Baby Care Basics

Dr. Jeremy Friedman, MB.ChB, FRCPC, FAAP,
Dr. Natasha Saunders, MD, MSc, FRCPC,
with Dr. Norman Saunders, MD, FRCPC

The Hospital for Sick Children

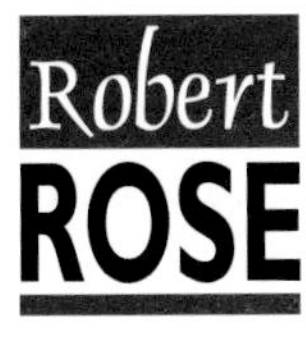

Robert ROSE

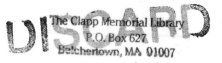

For a complete list of photo credits, see page 217.
For complete cataloguing information, see page 217.

Disclaimer

This book is a general guide only and should never be a substitute for the skill, knowledge and experience of a qualified medical professional dealing with the facts, circumstances and symptoms of a particular case.

The nutritional, medical, and health information presented in this book is based on the research, training, and professional experience of the authors, and is true and complete to the best of their knowledge. However, this book is intended only as an informative guide for those wishing to know more about health, nutrition, and medicine; it is not intended to replace or countermand the advice given by the reader's personal physician. Because each person and situation is unique, the authors and the publisher urge the reader to check with a qualified health-care professional before using any procedure where there is a question as to its appropriateness. The authors and the publisher are not responsible for any adverse effects or consequences resulting from the use of the information in this book. It is the responsibility of the reader to consult a physician or other qualified health-care professional regarding his or her personal care.

This book contains references to products that may not be available everywhere. The intent of the information provided is to be helpful; however, there is no guarantee of results associated with the information provided. Use of brand names is for educational purposes only and does not imply endorsement.

Design and production: Kevin Cockburn/PageWave Graphics Inc.
Editor: Sue Sumeraj
Proofreader: Kelly Jones
Indexer: Gillian Watts
Illustrations: Kveta/Three in a Box

The publisher gratefully acknowledges the financial support of our publishing program by the Government of Canada through the Canada Book Fund.

Published by Robert Rose Inc.
120 Eglinton Avenue East, Suite 800, Toronto, Ontario, Canada M4P 1E2
Tel: (416) 322-6552 Fax: (416) 322-6936
www.robertrose.ca

Printed and bound in Canada

1 2 3 4 5 6 7 8 9 TCP 23 22 21 20 19 18 17 16 15

To my husband, Justin Fluit;
my children, Nathan and Hailey Fluit; and
my parents, Lynn and Norman Saunders.

— NRS

To Shelley, Sam, and Dani, and
to my friend and mentor Norm Saunders,
who managed to get it so right.

— JF

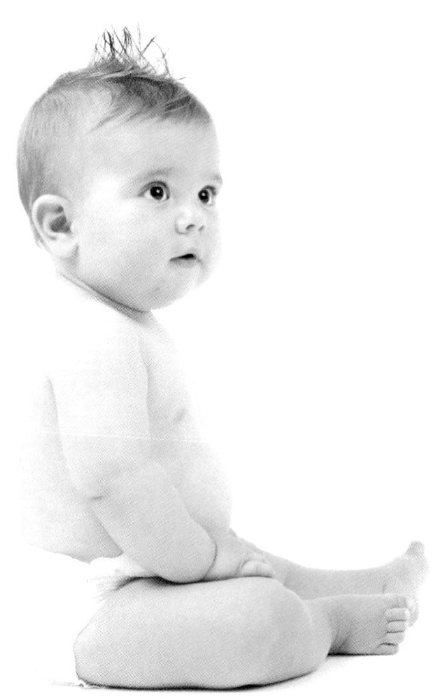

Contents

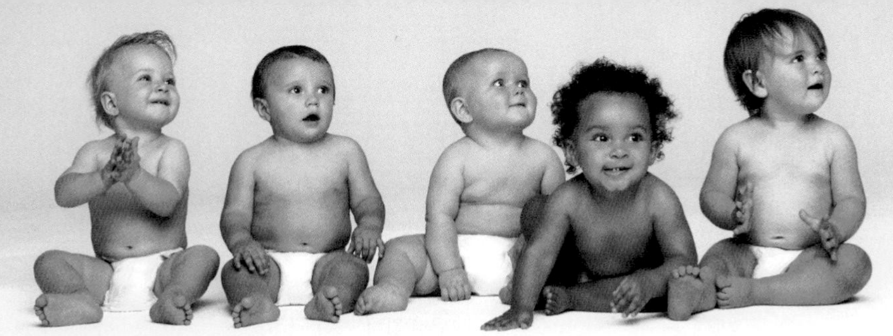

Introduction

DID YOU KNOW?

SICKKIDS HOSPITAL

SickKids is one of the top children's hospitals in the world and an iconic Canadian institution. For 140 years, parents have been bringing their children to SickKids for advice and treatment, and health-care providers come from across the world to be trained at this state of the art center. New discoveries are continually being made thanks to the innovative and very active research done by SickKids faculty.

Taking care of our children is one of life's biggest and most important challenges. We believe that, in general, parenting skills are intuitive and should not be overthought. That said, the right guide to the basics of taking care of a new baby can be extremely helpful, and many would consider it an essential tool for new parents.

Baby Care Basics is based on our comprehensive *Baby Care Book*, first published in 2007, which has helped many thousands of new parents from around the world. We compiled that book with the help of a group of top pediatricians at Toronto's SickKids hospital. Our contributors based their advice on the most up-to-date science as well as many years of experience looking after new babies and their families.

For this book, we extracted the most essential information and updated it based on current research and recommendations. Although there are many competing options in print or online to consult for advice in the care of your new baby, very few have the credibility and broad experience we have been able to tap into in compiling this book.

We have given you practical advice on everything you need to know from pregnancy through your baby's first year. In addition, we have devoted chapters to some of the areas we hear the most questions about as parents journey through the first year with a young infant: feeding, sleeping, safety, and illnesses.

We hope you will find the book easy to navigate and enjoyable, and that it answers the questions every new parent has on a daily basis. Congratulations on your new arrival. We wish you all the best in your adventures in parenting!

— Jeremy Friedman & Natasha Saunders

CHAPTER 1

Planning for a Baby

So you are planning for a new baby. Congratulations! You are about to embark on a wonderful journey that will enrich your life forever — probably even more than you can imagine. Most expectant parents wonder just how their lives will change with the arrival of their new baby. This time tends to be a mixture of anticipation, excitement, and some trepidation. There is no question that the addition of a new member to your family will require planning and adjustments to established routines.

Changes at Home

Accept the fact that you will need to adjust. Certainly your sleep patterns will be altered! However, the various changes that you, specifically, will experience with the arrival of a new baby will depend on many factors that are particular to you, your family, and your baby.

A baby's routines will change frequently throughout her first months. At first, it often seems that a newborn's only consistency is inconsistency! Flexibility and patience will be needed. While most new parents talk about their lives becoming busier with feeding, diapering, bathing, and washing their baby's clothes, some families find the initial days unexpectedly quiet, due to the considerable sleep requirements of a newborn.

New parents find that an activity or outing that used to be simple now requires planning and much more time than it did before. It is not unusual for any outing, such as a trip to the doctor for a checkup, to take half a day or more.

Everyone Has Advice

When you begin telling family, friends, and acquaintances that you are expecting a baby, you will probably find advice, invited and unsolicited, coming at you from all sides! While some advice can be helpful, many expectant parents find too much information stressful, overwhelming, or confusing. Remember, this experience is different for everyone. There is often no one right way of doing things.

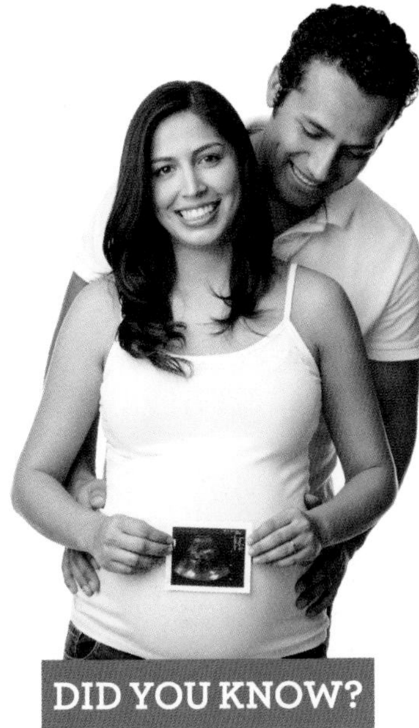

DID YOU KNOW?

SETTING PRIORITIES

If you have other children, you will be juggling several schedules. Planning becomes essential. Setting your priorities, focusing on those things you and your baby really need, and leaving less important tasks undone will help. Vacuuming can probably wait for another day ... or even week.

HOW TO: Prepare Siblings for a New Baby

Children, even young ones, tend to know when any significant change is occurring in their lives. You need to prepare them for the arrival of a new member of the family. Besides, they should be included in the excitement and anticipation you are experiencing!

Siblings adjust better to an approaching birth if they have an understanding of what is happening. How you tell your children about the impending new arrival will depend on their age and level of understanding:

For young siblings, talking about "the baby in Mommy's tummy" is appropriate. Allowing them to feel the baby move or kick will make the anticipated arrival more real.

For older children, make them feel part of the experience by involving them in planning. Discussing ways they can help once the baby arrives will make them feel included.

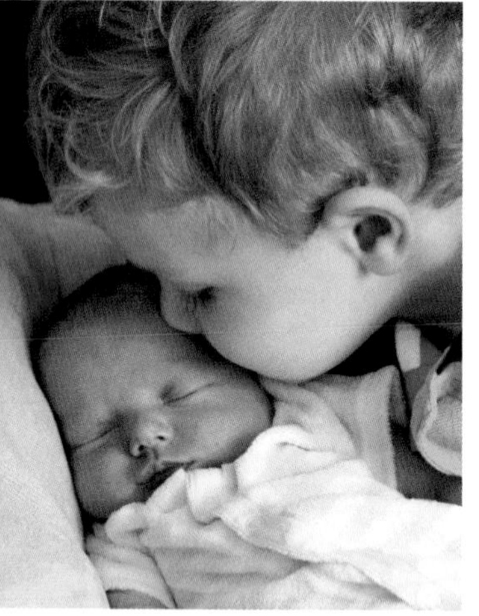

Don't be afraid to change the subject or tune out if you have had enough. You will also want to develop a good relationship with your health-care provider, who will see you through your pregnancy and your baby's birth.

Health-Care Options

One of the first decisions you need to make involves choosing the health-care professional who will monitor your pregnancy and assist with your baby's birth. There are several options, including a family doctor, a midwife, or an obstetrician. Your choice is an individual decision, based on your family's preferences and health histories. Whichever option you choose, it is important for expectant mothers to be examined regularly to ensure that any problems are addressed promptly. You should make this decision as early as possible and set up an appointment with your health-care provider to discuss the next steps.

Tests and More Tests

A number of screening tests are typically done during a pregnancy to monitor the fetus and assess the expectant mother for conditions that might affect the baby's health at birth and beyond. At each visit to your health-care provider, your weight and the size of your uterus will be measured to ensure that the baby is growing appropriately. The baby's heartbeat will be assessed using a small ultrasound probe placed on your abdomen. Your blood pressure and urine will also be checked.

Common Tests During Pregnancy

TEST NAME	TIMING	WHY?
Blood group and antibody screen (blood)	1st trimester	Differences between your and your baby's blood type may lead to severe jaundice (yellow discoloration of the skin) in your baby shortly after delivery.
Hepatitis B surface antigen (blood)	1st trimester	If you or a household member has this liver disease, your baby will require immunization immediately after birth.
HIV antibody (blood)	1st trimester	Early detection and treatment with antiviral medication can lead to a huge reduction in the risk of transmission of HIV to the baby.
Rubella immunity (blood)	1st trimester	To check if you have immunity to rubella (German measles). Rubella acquired during pregnancy can lead to a number of birth defects. Unimmunized mothers require a vaccine just after delivery.
VDRL (blood)	1st trimester	To test for syphilis, which could be present without symptoms. Early detection and treatment with antibiotics is critical to ensure delivery of a healthy baby.
Pre-eclampsia test (blood pressure and urine test)	At each visit	High blood pressure with protein in the urine during pregnancy can mean the baby may need to be delivered earlier than expected.
Diabetes screen (blood)	24 to 28 weeks gestation	High sugar levels can indicate diabetes. Treatment throughout pregnancy is required, often through a combination of dietary changes or medication to ensure the best outcomes for the baby.
Ultrasound	12 to 13 weeks and 18 to 20 weeks	Ultrasounds assess the size and growth of the fetus, enable visualization of the placenta's placement in the uterus, and provide a picture of the baby's body structures.
Group B streptococcus (GBS) (rectal and vaginal swab)	35 to 37 weeks	This bacteria is found in approximately 10% to 30% of pregnant women. While harmless to a mom, GBS can infect the baby's bloodstream, resulting in serious illness. Antibiotics are given to infected mothers after their water breaks, prior to delivery, to help prevent transmission to the baby.

Special Tests

A number of specialized screening tests for potential congenital malformations or genetic disorders in the fetus may be offered or be available to you. Examples include screening for spina bifida and screening for trisomy 21 (Down syndrome). The need for these will depend on your personal and family health history, age, and pregnancy history.

Other screening tests for rare diseases, such as Tay-Sachs disease or cystic fibrosis, may be suggested, particularly if your ethnic background suggests a greater risk for such conditions.

Amniocentesis, which tests the amniotic fluid surrounding the baby, or chorionic villus sampling from the growing placenta, may be recommended, depending on your family's health history and risk factors. Recent technological advances analyzing fetal DNA in a mother's blood are now being used to detect some genetic abnormalities as early as 10 weeks into a pregnancy.

DID YOU KNOW?

TO TEST OR NOT TO TEST?

Some families wish to have all of the specialized screening tests, and others do not. Consider whether knowing the results will help you prepare better for your baby's birth or will make a difference in your decision to continue the pregnancy.

Eating for Two

Although it does not justify overeating or overindulging food cravings, there is some truth in the old expression that you are now "eating for two." As your pregnancy progresses, your nutrient requirements increase. Balanced consumption of the three macronutrients — carbohydrate, protein, and fat — will provide you with the energy you need to feed the two of you, while supplementation of the key micronutrients — calcium, vitamin D, folic acid, iron, and zinc — will promote the general health of mother and child during pregnancy and after delivery. Before making any changes to your diet, be sure to consult your health-care provider or a dietitian registered with the American Dietetic Association or the Dietitians of Canada.

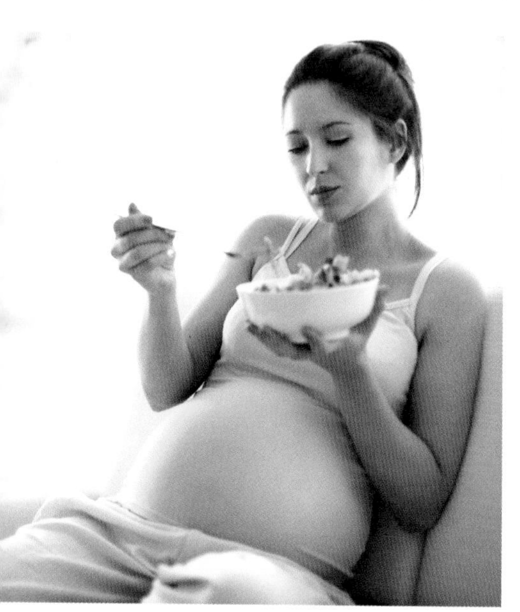

Energy Needs

During the first trimester, your energy needs will increase by 100 calories a day, and during the second and third trimester, by 300 calories a day, to an optimum 2,200 to 2,700 calories, spread across three meals and one or two snacks.

Daily Recommended Intake of Nutrients During Pregnancy

CARBOHYDRATE	PROTEIN	FAT	CALCIUM
175 g	71 g	20%–35% of total energy intake	1000 mg

VITAMIN D	FOLIC ACID	IRON	ZINC
600 IU	600 mcg	27 mg	11 mg

Adapted with permission from Daina Kalnins and Joanne Saab, *Better Food for Pregnancy* (Toronto: Robert Rose, 2006).

Special Nutrient Requirements

Several specific minerals and vitamins are needed to ensure a healthy pregnancy. These nutrients can be obtained from food sources, but you may need to take a supplement.

Adequate calcium and vitamin D are essential for the healthy growth and development of the fetus. Folic acid, taken as a supplement before you become pregnant and until the end of the first trimester, can reduce the risk of neural tube defects, such as spina bifida. Iron is crucial, because an iron deficiency can lower immunity and increase the risk of infection and illness.

Planning a Safe and Healthy Pregnancy

Planning is a big part of a successful pregnancy. You will want to think about everything from your emotional readiness for raising a child to more immediate concerns about finding the right caregiver after your baby is born. Even before you become pregnant, you will want to decrease your risk of exposure to known teratogens — medications, chemicals, and infections that can cause birth defects.

If your pregnancy is not planned, don't worry. Nearly half of all pregnancies are unplanned, and the vast majority of children born in North America are normal and healthy. Still, you'll want to get the facts from the experts on the do's and don'ts of exposure to drugs and other substances.

In the meantime, on the following pages you'll find 10 steps to a safe and healthy pregnancy.

DID YOU KNOW?

FOOD GUIDES

One of the best ways to ensure a healthy diet before, during, and after pregnancy is to follow the nutritional advice in the United States Department of Agriculture's MyPlate guidelines (choosemyplate.gov) or in Eating Well with Canada's Food Guide (www.hc-sc.gc.ca/fn-an/food-guide-aliment/index-eng.php).

10 Steps for a Healthy Pregnancy

1. **Take folic acid to prevent neural tube defects and other congenital anomalies.** Folic acid is vital for the body when cells are growing and multiplying rapidly. With sufficient amounts of folic acid in your diet and through dietary supplementation, you dramatically decrease the risk of spina bifida. Neural tube defects are major congenital anomalies of the brain or spinal cord that occur when the brain or spine fails to close properly. This crucial event occurs very early in pregnancy — so early, in fact, that many women run the risk of a neural tube defect before they even know they have conceived.

   Folic acid is one of the B vitamins, found naturally in green, leafy vegetables, nuts, and oranges. In North America, flour is fortified with folic acid, so it is present in breads and pastas. However, a healthy pregnancy requires 400 to 1000 micrograms of folic acid every day, a quantity many women may not get through diet alone. All women should start taking a daily prenatal multivitamin before becoming pregnant. This will ensure adequate amounts of folic acid for healthy fetal development. Most pregnancy multivitamin tablets contain around 1000 micrograms of folic acid.

2. **Stop drinking alcohol to prevent fetal alcohol spectrum disorder.** Fetal alcohol spectrum disorder (FASD) is the leading cause of preventable brain damage, caused by the developing brain's exposure to alcohol. Women often ask if there is a safe amount of alcohol they can drink during pregnancy. The answer is, we just don't know. That's why the most prudent choice when planning your pregnancy is to avoid alcohol entirely. If avoiding alcohol is a challenge for you, ask your health-care provider for help.

3. **Stop smoking cigarettes to help prevent stillbirth, prematurity, and sudden infant death syndrome.** When planning a pregnancy, you should stop smoking. Smoking in pregnancy may decrease the baby's birth weight and increase the risk of stillbirth (fetal death after 20 weeks of gestation) and prematurity (baby born before 37 weeks of pregnancy). It also increases your risk for miscarriage. In addition, smoking in

DID YOU KNOW?

PLANNING FOR PREGNANCY

Planning your pregnancy and taking folic acid supplements before conception and multivitamins throughout pregnancy, for 4 to 6 weeks after delivery, and as long as you are breast-feeding will ensure that your child is protected, especially in those very early days of development.

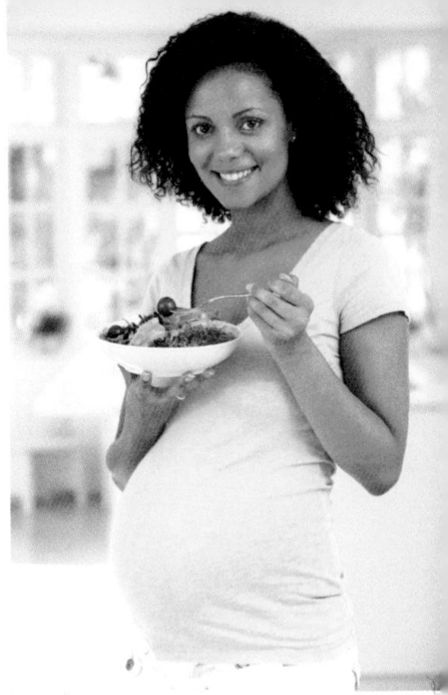

pregnancy is associated with sudden infant death syndrome (SIDS), or "crib death," where infants die during their sleep for no apparent reason. If you're having trouble kicking the habit, think about getting help. Talk to your doctor. Nicotine replacement therapy (nicotine patch, gum, or spray) or Zyban (bupropion) tablets may be right for you. Both methods have been shown in controlled randomized trials to be effective in smoking cessation.

4. **Treat drug dependencies.** If you are dependent on or addicted to prescription medications, such as morphine or oxycodone, or to recreational drugs, such as cocaine or marijuana, seek addiction counseling and treatment before pregnancy. Drug dependencies or abuse may affect your baby directly by entering the baby's body or indirectly by affecting your health and/or your ability to care for your baby. Remember that drug dependency is not limited to the use of "street drugs" but may also involve common medications, such as pain relievers. If "kicking the habit" is a challenge for you, ask your health-care provider for help.
5. **Immunize against preventable infectious diseases.** When planning your pregnancy, you should ensure that you are immunized against viruses that are dangerous for the unborn baby. Rubella is one virus that some women may have lost their immunity to, despite being appropriately vaccinated in childhood. Similarly, some women may have never had chicken pox (varicella) or been immunized against the virus. You can get the vaccine from your doctor if a blood test shows that you are not immune.

   The annual influenza vaccine (flu shot) is helpful for pregnant women, to protect both the mother and her fetus from catching the flu, which can be especially dangerous for young babies, who cannot be vaccinated before the age of 6 months.
6. **Seek proper treatment of medical conditions.** If you have a chronic medical condition, this is the time to ensure that you are treated with medications that are safe for the fetus. Discuss with your health-care provider whether pregnancy will affect your medical condition, and whether your medical condition will affect the pregnancy.

KEY POINT

The influenza vaccine is safe and effective during pregnancy. Make sure you get your annual flu shot to protect yourself, your fetus, and your infant after delivery.

Don't stop medications "cold turkey." Many medications do not pose a risk to the fetus. What's more, if you have relied on certain prescription medications to control conditions such as hypertension or depression, you may do more harm than good by suddenly stopping your medication. You can often continue your medication during pregnancy, but your doctor may want to prescribe an alternative, safer medication. Remember that many untreated conditions themselves pose a risk to the fetus.

7. **Do not self-prescribe.** You may be used to treating your coughs, colds, aches, and pains with one or more of the products for sale at your local drugstore, but once you are pregnant (or planning a pregnancy), over-the-counter self-help must end. What is safe for you may not be safe for your fetus. Be particularly cautious with the use of herbal medicines — there is little human data on their safety or risk in pregnancy.
8. **Avoid exposure to dangerous chemicals in the workplace.** If your occupation involves exposure to chemicals, find out which ones are involved and seek advice on their safety for your developing fetus. Exposure to chemical solvents and heavy metals can pose a risk to your baby. The ones you have likely heard the most about are carbon monoxide, formaldehyde, lead, mercury, and organic solvents, but there are others.
9. **Seek preconception genetic counseling.** If you or your partner has a family history of children born with congenital malformations or developmental delays (your own children or those of your siblings), your health-care provider can refer you for genetic counseling, which usually involves a detailed assessment of your medical, obstetric, and family history.
10. **Be confident.** There is plenty of excellent, evidence-based information to guide you through your pregnancy and while you breast-feed your child. Your health-care providers are there to help. Ask questions and learn the facts. The list of known teratogens (medications, chemicals, and infections that have been proven unsafe to an unborn baby) is relatively short. The list of substances that are not compatible with breast-feeding is even shorter. Stay informed, and your odds of having a safe pregnancy and a healthy baby are excellent.

DID YOU KNOW?

TERATOGEN INFORMATION SERVICES

Organization of Teratogen Information Services (OTIS)

For local teratogen information services in most states and provinces in North America, contact OTIS at (866) 626-6847. Information about OTIS is also available at www.mothertobaby.org.

Motherisk

The Motherisk Program at the Hospital for Sick Children in Toronto is one of the largest teratogen counseling and education centers in the world. Contact Motherisk at (877) 439-2744 or at www.motherisk.org.

GUIDE TO: Medications That Are Safe and Unsafe in Pregnancy

A number of medications have been associated with fetal malformations or problems with development. If you believe you have been exposed to these potential teratogens before or during pregnancy, contact your health-care provider immediately. This list is by no means exhaustive but represents a few of the commonly used medications. For more detailed information, contact OTIS or Motherisk (see sidebar, page 14).

Medications Generally Considered SAFE in Pregnancy

- Acetaminophen
- Acyclovir
- Amoxicillin
- Calcium carbonate (Tums)
- Cephalosporin antibiotics
- Diphenhydramine (Benadryl)
- Loratadine (Claritin)
- Nitrofurantoin (Macrobid)
- Ranitidine (Zantac)
- Saline nasal spay

Medications Generally Considered UNSAFE in Pregnancy

- Accutane
- Anti-cancer medications
- Aspirin
- Bismuth subsalicylate (Pepto-Bismol)
- Carbamazepine (Tegretol)
- Corticosteroids (by mouth)
- Nonsteroidal anti-inflammatory drugs (NSAIDs), such as ibuprofen (Advil/Motrin)
- Phenytoin (Dilantin)
- Tetracycline
- Valproic acid
- Warfarin

Choosing Your Baby's Doctor

Before your baby is born, you should choose a health-care provider to follow your baby's growth and development after birth. You may choose to have your own family doctor, a pediatrician, a nurse, or a health clinic care for your baby. Some pediatricians, who are specialists in child health, do "well baby" visits, while others only follow children with health problems. Here are some points to consider when making your decision.

KEY POINT

Identify a health-care provider for your baby *before* you deliver to ensure that you have help in place should your baby have any health concerns immediately after she leaves the hospital.

1. **Convenience:** During the first months, frequent visits are required to monitor your baby's growth and development, so having a care provider close to where you live may be important.
2. **Comfort:** Pick someone you trust and with whom you feel comfortable asking questions. Ask family members

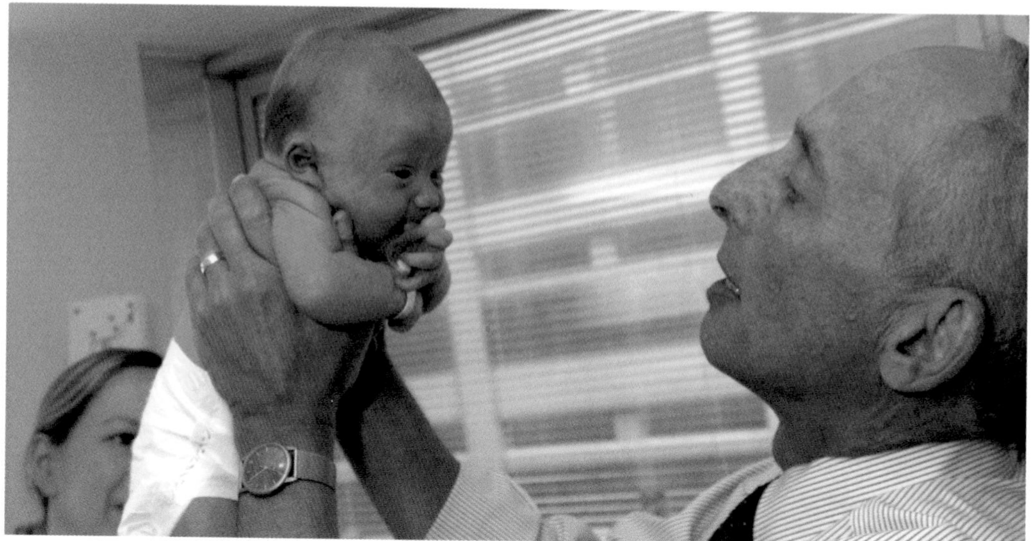

and friends for their advice. Your own doctor may also have recommendations.

3. **Accessibility:** If you have a concern about your baby's health at night or on a weekend, how will you get help? How is the practice set up — is it a solo practice or a partnership of practitioners who share on-call duty?

What Will Your Baby Need?

There is an overwhelming selection of baby products awaiting you. Despite changes in fashion and technical advances, the paramount concern is still safety.

Initially, your baby's needs are simple: a place to eat, a place to sleep, a place to have her diapers changed, and a place to be bathed. If you want to be mobile, you'll also need a safe means of transportation. Here is a guide to meeting these basic needs.

A Place to Eat

You will spend considerable time feeding your baby, so you might as well be comfortable. Create a peaceful place where you and your baby can feel relaxed. Of course, if you have other children, this is easier said than done.

Many parents choose a simple rocking chair or a glider rocker (a particular favorite due to its smooth rocking motion), but any comfortable chair with a cushioned seat, footrest, and armrests will do. Place a table beside your chair to keep a glass of water, a damp cloth, reading material, and a phone close by.

A Place to Sleep

You will need to decide where your baby will spend her first days at home. Some parents choose to have the newborn sleep in their room, while others prefer to have a dedicated baby's room. Some parents prefer a bassinet, some a crib. Others prefer to co-sleep with their newborn.

Bassinets

Some families choose to use a bassinet initially. However, your baby will very quickly outgrow a bassinet and require a larger sleeping space. Be aware of safety issues — some bassinets have handles, allowing transport of a sleeping baby from room to room, but the bassinet can easily be dropped by a tired parent. Others attach to the side of an adult bed, but care must be taken to ensure that there is no gap or possibility of entrapment between beds.

KEY POINT

Never place your baby to sleep on a couch — there is a risk of suffocation.

Cribs

Many parents choose to have their baby sleep in a crib. If you are buying a new crib, look for a product certification from a reputable testing agency. If you are planning to use a second-hand or older crib, make sure it meets current safety standards. For example, sides that slide up and down are no longer considered safe due to risk of injury. The National Safety Council (www.nsc.org) and the Consumer Product Safety Commission (www.cpsc.gov) provide guides to these safety standards.

DID YOU KNOW?

CO-SLEEPING

Some families plan to co-sleep with their newborn for ease of nursing. Be cautious if you do so. Co-sleeping with adults who are obese, overtired (most new parents!), or under the influence of alcohol or drugs may be associated with a higher risk of sudden infant death syndrome (SIDS).

Safe Bedding

The mattress you use should be approved for newborns. It should be firm, not soft. Use only a thin or porous blanket and do not give your baby a pillow. The current recommendation is that infants sleep on their backs. Sleep positioners (wedges used to prop a baby on her side) are not recommended, and some may pose a suffocation risk.

Strollers

Your choice of stroller should be based on where you intend to use it; the weather conditions in your area; whether you intend to take it in the car or on a plane; the number of young children you have; and, of course, price restrictions. You will likely use your stroller for a few years, so durability is another important factor.

DID YOU KNOW?

BABY CARRIERS

Some caregivers prefer to carry their young infants in an infant carrier or "snuggly." There are several brands on the market and many different styles. Try them out and pick the one that feels most comfortable and secure. As your child gets heavier, a carrier with good back support will be helpful.

DID YOU KNOW?

DISPOSABLE OR WASHABLE?

Disposable diapers are convenient, particularly for use out of the home. And rashes are less likely with disposable diapers than with cloth diapers. However, disposable diapers are expensive and environmentally unfriendly, creating a significant amount of garbage. Cloth diapers are reusable but must be changed promptly to avoid diaper rashes. You may choose to wash them yourself or use a diaper service, which picks up soiled diapers and replaces them with new ones.

The many strollers on the market differ in size and weight, the number of wheels, the suspension, the folding mechanism, the available storage area, and the number of seats. Several models allow you to clamp your car seat onto the frame of the stroller so you don't have to move your sleeping baby. If you choose this option, ensure that the car seat and the stroller are compatible. The car seat must be securely clamped in place when attached to the stroller.

If you have more than one child, there are various double strollers available. Tandem strollers (one child seated in front of the other) are easier to maneuver in public places, but are large and heavy. Side-by-side strollers are another option. They look pretty wide, but they do fit through most doorways.

A Place to Have Diapers Changed

If there is one thing your baby will require frequently, it is diaper changes! You will need a stable, clean surface for this job. Some parents use a blanket or change pad on the floor. A portable change pad to take with you for diaper changes outside your home is especially handy.

Many parents opt to purchase or borrow a change table. The advantage of change tables is their comfortable height. The disadvantage is that babies can wiggle or roll off change tables if you're not watching. Be sure to keep a hand on your baby at all times. Place the necessities for diaper changing (diapers, cream, and wipes) within reach.

A Place to Be Bathed

Many new parents choose to purchase a baby bathtub rather than use the adult tub or the sink for bathing their baby. Keep several small facecloths around to wipe your baby's hands and face while bathing and after eating. Mild baby soap can be used to wash your baby's skin and hair.

Diaper Bags

As you become more mobile, it will be helpful to have a diaper bag ready to go with supplies for the road. Select a bag that can hold a few diapers, wipes, a small change pad, a change of baby clothes, and a blanket or burp cloth. It's a good idea to have a small insulated bottle bag, which can hold bottles of expressed breast milk or formula. Later, you can use this to carry baby food and a "sippy" cup.

Car Seats

There is considerable evidence that infants and children are safest in cars when they are secured in special child car seats. Car seats should be placed in the back seat. Car seats that are used until the child is at least 40 pounds (18 kg) have an internal seat belt that fastens the child to the seat. They are secured to the vehicle's seat using the vehicle seat belt or a "LATCH" Universal Anchorage System (metal clips secured to the car frame).

Your child's car seat must be placed properly in your car and held tightly in place as recommended by the seat and car manufacturers. The internal seat belt must be tightened properly, leaving a maximum of one finger width between the chest clip and your child's body, with the chest clip at the level of your child's underarms. In many larger centers, professionals can check the seat installation for you — ask about this service when you purchase your car seat.

In general, there are three stages of car seat requirements for children: those for newborns and infants; those for toddlers; and those for school-age children. There are combination seats and convertible seats that may cover two to three of these stages, but they are generally more expensive. Choose the car seat that fits most securely into your vehicle.

KEY POINT

The front seat is not safe for children until they are at least 13 years old because of the presence of air bags, which may cause significant injuries to a child when activated.

KEY POINT

Car seats are essential to ensure the safety of your infant or child, but they are only effective if properly fitted and secured according to the manufacturer's instructions.

1. **Newborns and infants:** Because newborns and young infants have poor head control, they require a seat that is relatively reclined. This style of seat must be used until your baby reaches 22 pounds (10 kg), 1 year of age, and is walking. The seat is placed in the vehicle with the infant facing the rear of the car, permitting maximal head support in the event of a crash. The seat can be secured directly to the car using the car seat belt or clipped into a base that remains in the car and is secured by the car's seat belt or using a Universal Anchorage System. This type of car seat has a handle that can be raised or lowered, and the baby can be carried outside the vehicle within the car seat. If your child reaches 22 pounds (10 kg) or is walking before 1 year of age, she can be moved up to a toddler car seat, but should remain facing the rear.

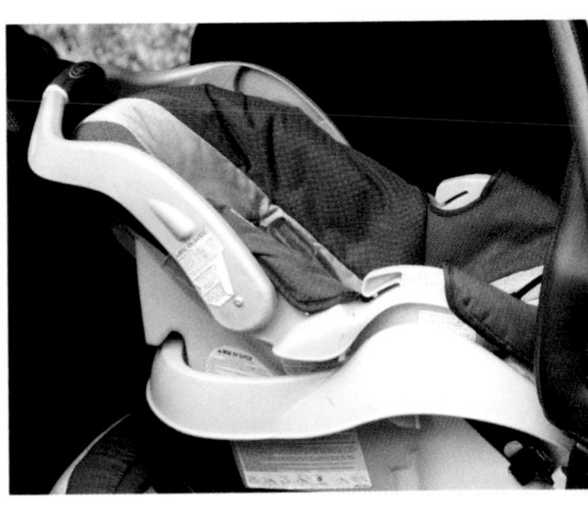

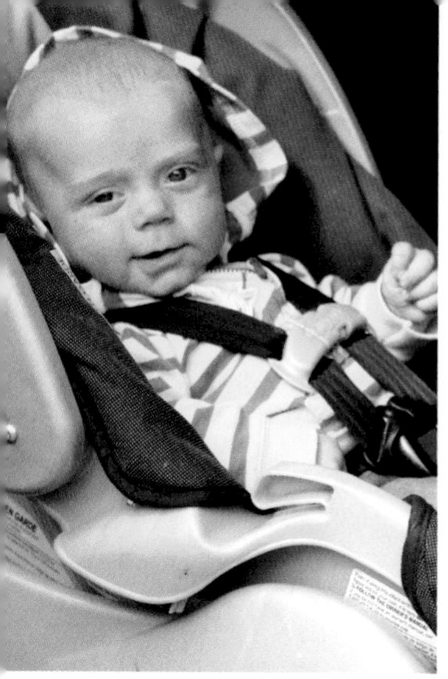

2. **Toddlers:** Once your child reaches 22 pounds (10 kg), 1 year of age, and is walking, she may be seated in a toddler car seat; however, the American Academy of Pediatrics and the Canadian Paediatric Society recommend keeping your child facing the rear as long as possible, providing she meets the car seat manufacturer's guidelines for height and weight restrictions. In the United States, recommendations state that a child should continue facing the rear window until 2 years of age. From this point until she reaches 40 pounds (18 kg), at approximately 4 years of age, your child should remain in a toddler seat. This type of seat is placed in an upright position and contains an internal seat belt. To protect your child from injury, the seat must be secured tightly to the car frame using the car's seat belt or with a Universal Anchorage System.
3. **School-age children:** Once she reaches 40 pounds (18 kg), and until she reaches 80 pounds (36 kg) and 145 cm (4 feet, 9 inches), at about 8 years of age, your child should remain in a "booster" seat to protect against lower spinal cord injuries. A booster seat has no internal seat belt, but simply raises the child slightly to allow the vehicle's seat belt to be positioned properly over the hips. Shoulder strap positioners allow the belt to be positioned comfortably and safely over the shoulder. Booster seats do not require tethering to the car frame.

KEY POINT

You may want to prepare and freeze some meals ahead of time: you're unlikely to find much time to cook in your first week at home.

Getting Ready for the Delivery

Once you have decided where the birth will take place, you may want to arrange a visit to familiarize yourself with where to go. Start packing everything you will want to take to the hospital or birthing center — for your own needs and your baby's needs.

What to Pack

FOR YOU	FOR BABY
• Underwear, nursing bra • Comfortable, loose, dark clothing • "Overnight" pads • Slippers or comfortable shoes • Some favorite foods, snacks, and drinks • Phone and camera	• Newborn-size diapers, wipes, and petroleum jelly • Clothing appropriate for the weather, including a hat • Blanket • Car seat, if you plan to drive home

Frequently Asked Questions

As pediatricians, we answer many questions from parents. At the end of each chapter in this book are some of the most frequently asked questions. Be sure to ask your health-care providers any other questions that arise. If they don't have the answers, they will refer you to a colleague who does.

Everybody thinks I'm going to have a girl. What is the best test to predict the sex of my baby?

There are a lot of popular myths, theories, and old wives' tales that claim the ability to predict a baby's sex. How you are "carrying" your baby, whether you have indigestion, and many other signs have been put forward as trustworthy indications of fetal sex. But the only reliable way to determine the sex of your child is to have a health-care provider examine the genitals on an ultrasound, test the chromosomes in a sample of amniotic fluid taken by amniocentesis, or do a blood test to look for cell-free fetal DNA in maternal blood. Discuss with your partner whether you really want to know — it is a very personal decision. If your answer is yes, ask your health-care provider to check for you.

My husband is adamant that our baby boy be circumcised. My reading suggests that it is better to leave the foreskin alone. This is one of our first decisions as parents, and I want to get it right ... without a fight. What should I do?

Parents often disagree about what is best for their child. Now is as good a time as any to establish some general guidelines on how you, as a couple, will handle these disagreements. For starters, it's best to review the facts involved in this or any issue. A little extra information can sometimes be quite persuasive. Then, see if there is some strong emotional reason behind the adamant viewpoint.

Circumcision involves the surgical removal of the foreskin covering the head of the penis. This procedure is relatively simple, with few complications, although it can be painful, and there is a small risk of bleeding, infection, and poor healing. Pain reduction should be a regular part of the circumcision procedure. One method involves injecting freezing around the nerve supplying the penis. This works in a similar way to the technique used by dentists to "freeze" teeth. Not all doctors will perform circumcisions, and there might be an additional cost for the procedure.

While circumcised boys have a lower incidence of urinary tract infections and less risk later in life of developing penile cancer and some sexually transmitted diseases, such as HIV, there is no overwhelming advantage to circumcision, so the decision is an individual one based on your religious or personal preference.

Do your best to understand your partner's position. You would be surprised at the number of men who want their son to look just like them. A little extra skin should be no big deal. Try to retain your sense of humor. If the issue is still unresolved after forthright discussion, meet with your health-care provider, who can help mediate the dispute.

I have heard about cord blood banking. Is this a good idea?

There is no simple answer to this question. Since the first cord blood banking service started in 1991, many programs have been created to collect blood from the umbilical cord at the time of delivery and store it for potential transplantation at a later stage. Some programs are funded by large not-for-profit organizations, such as the National Institutes of Health and the American Red Cross, while others are private for-profit businesses. In most not-for-profit programs, the cord blood collected is available to anyone who needs it and is a "match," while the for-profit businesses encourage parents to bank their infant's cord blood as a form of "biological insurance" for their own private use.

No accurate estimates exist of the probability that children will need their own stored cord blood cells in the future (estimates range from one in 1,000 to one in 200,000). While cord blood has been shown to be curative in some individual patients with a number of serious genetic, blood, cancer, and immune disorders, the evidence of its safety or effectiveness for the treatment of cancer in the child (donor) at a later stage remains unclear.

The latest recommendation from the American Academy of Pediatrics is that cord blood donation should be discouraged if it is to be directed for later personal or family use (biological insurance) because most conditions that might be helped by cord blood stem cells already exist in the infant's cord blood. However, if a sibling in the family has a known condition that may potentially benefit from cord blood transplantation, directed cord blood banking should be encouraged. Cord blood donation should also be encouraged when the cord blood is stored in a bank for public use, but parents need to realize that this blood may not be accessible in the future for private use.

If you wish to have your baby's cord blood collected, you must give your consent in writing. The procedure is not painful for you or for your baby. The blood is taken from the umbilical cord, which would otherwise normally be discarded. Arrangements must be made prior to your delivery so that appropriate cord blood collection and storage equipment is available.

Getting ready for our new baby seems to require making a lot of purchases. With my wife starting maternity leave, how will we be able to afford all these necessary items?

Truthfully, parenting is never cheap, nor does it come without sacrifice. Kids have expensive needs at all ages: first, tons of diapers; then, lots of outfits; next, sports equipment and music lessons; and later, college tuition. Fortunately, we can convince ourselves that it is all worthwhile.

Like all projects, preparing for a new baby requires budgeting. If you are joggers, you might choose to splurge on a special stroller, but that might mean the rocking chair in the nursery comes from a garage sale. As long as your purchases meet the safety code, used or less expensive items are just fine.

Friends and relatives are always trying to find the perfect baby gift. A tactful suggestion or a creative partnership can transform a less wanted teddy bear into the change table you really need.

Finally, it's important to remind yourselves that the happiest children aren't always the ones with the most expensive stuff: as the song suggests, love is all you really need.

CHAPTER 2

Your Baby's First Few Days

You've spent months anticipating your baby's arrival, daydreaming about life with your baby and making plans for your family's future. The nursery is painted, the receiving blankets are folded, and the car seat is installed. But if this is your first child, you may not have considered what exactly will happen during the first few moments of your baby's life. Who will be present in the delivery room to help out with this amazing transition? How will your baby react as he moves from the comfort and warmth of the womb to the strange air-breathing world? If anything goes wrong, what can be done?

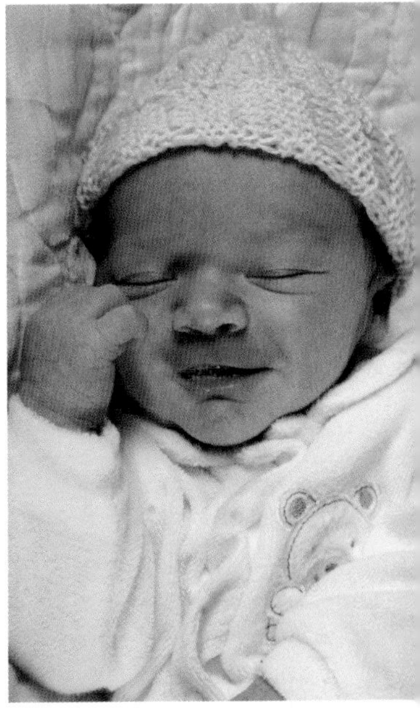

Delivering Your Baby

This is a short, exciting, and crucial time. What exactly takes place will differ depending on the setting in which you've chosen to deliver and the ease with which your labor has progressed.

Who Will Be Present?

By now, you have probably decided on the people you would like with you in the delivery room. Besides your personal choices, the faces in the delivery room will largely depend on the setting in which you have chosen to give birth.

Midwife

If a midwife will be attending your delivery, she will likely be at your side throughout the active stages of labor, working with you to deliver your baby and attending afterwards to both of your needs.

Family Doctor "On Call"

Alternatively, you might choose your family doctor to serve a similar role. Increasingly, family physicians work as part of a larger group who rotate being "on call" for deliveries. In this scenario, one of your doctor's trusted colleagues may deliver your baby. Your prenatal records will be available, of course, to the physician on call.

DID YOU KNOW?

ASK QUESTIONS

Remember that it is your right to know the role of everyone in the delivery room, so if they do not introduce themselves, be sure to ask. Regardless of how your birthing center is run, you should be confident that team members are specialists and know their own skills and limitations. It is best to discuss any questions or concerns you might have early on.

Obstetrician

The most common option in North America is to have an obstetrician — a surgeon who specializes in delivering babies — attend you. If yours is a complicated situation, the obstetrician may be consulted by your midwife or family physician to provide expertise and help you with the delivery.

> **DID YOU KNOW?**
>
> **NO COMPLICATIONS**
>
> If your labor progresses without complication, do not be surprised if the physician on call is not present until the last minute, to aid in the baby's delivery.

Nurses

Labor and delivery nurses are an integral part of the birthing process. One specific nurse will usually be assigned to you and will follow your progress in the labor and delivery room. This nurse is often the key to good communication, as she will liaise between you and the other health-care professionals. If you have specific requests or wishes about your labor and delivery experience, make sure to inform your nurse.

Respiratory Therapist

Respiratory therapists are often part of the health-care team, particularly at larger centers. They are experts in the baby's airway and breathing. At some hospitals, they attend each birth; at others, they are called when needed, to ensure that your baby's lungs are adapting appropriately to the air-breathing world.

> **DID YOU KNOW?**
>
> **EXPECT THE UNEXPECTED**
>
> No matter how well you try to prepare yourself for labor and delivery, it will remain somewhat unpredictable. Like so much in your baby's first year of life, there will be some things out of your control. You will need to be flexible in your approach. Rest assured that the team you have assembled will have the expertise to guide you on a safe journey into parenthood.

Pediatrician

Pediatricians are often called to attend deliveries if there are problems that arise just prior to, at, or immediately following the delivery. They are present so that someone with a high level of expertise in newborn care is there, dedicated to ensuring that your baby transitions into the real world as safely as possible. For example, pediatricians routinely attend deliveries for twins and premature babies, or if there are signs during labor that your baby may be in distress.

Anesthesiologist

Last but not least, an anesthesiologist, a physician with expertise in pain control, will follow your case. The anesthesiologist can help reduce the discomfort of a vaginal birth or provide anesthesia in the event a Caesarian section is required. Pain control is usually achieved with an epidural or, more rarely, with a general anesthetic.

Induction of Labor

Some women may not go into labor spontaneously, or, when they do, the labor may progress very slowly. Health-care providers may need to induce or augment labor to protect the health of the baby and the mother. Three ways to do this include ripening the cervix with a vaginal insert, intravenous medications to start uterine contractions, or breaking the membrane that encircles the baby and amniotic fluid.

Indications for Induction

- The pregnancy has gone past 41 weeks, and there is concern about the placenta's ability to provide adequate oxygen and nutrition to the baby.
- You have high blood pressure or diabetes, which could harm you or your baby.
- You have a uterine infection.
- Your waters have broken, but contractions haven't begun.

Breech Babies

Although many babies are "heads-up" early in the pregnancy, most of them will rotate into a head-down position in the mother's uterus prior to delivery — which is why the head emerges first. If the baby has his head up and either his buttocks or feet pointing down close to the time of delivery, this is called the breech position.

If your health-care provider suspects that the baby is in a breech position, this can be confirmed by ultrasound. Most doctors prefer to deliver breech babies by Caesarian section because they consider it safer for the baby. In select cases, doctors may try to turn the baby in the mother's uterus, using a procedure called external cephalic version.

Caesarian Section

A Caesarian section (C-section) refers to the delivery of the baby through a surgical incision made in the mother's lower abdominal wall and uterus. This is generally done by a specialist (an obstetrician). Rates vary among different jurisdictions, but in North America, roughly 30% of deliveries are now by C-section.

In some cases, your health-care provider may recommend that an elective, or planned, C-section be performed before you have a chance to go into labor on your own. Other times, if there are concerns during labor that the

DID YOU KNOW?

FETAL MONITORING IN LABOR

During labor, your baby's well-being will be closely observed, which generally involves monitoring the fetal heart rate as well as your uterine contractions through a very sensitive ultrasound probe attached to your abdomen with a belt. A gel, which often feels cold, is used to help conduct the ultrasound signal to and from the fetus. The fetal heart rate usually varies between 100 and 160 beats a minute. Your heart rate, blood pressure, and temperature will also be closely observed.

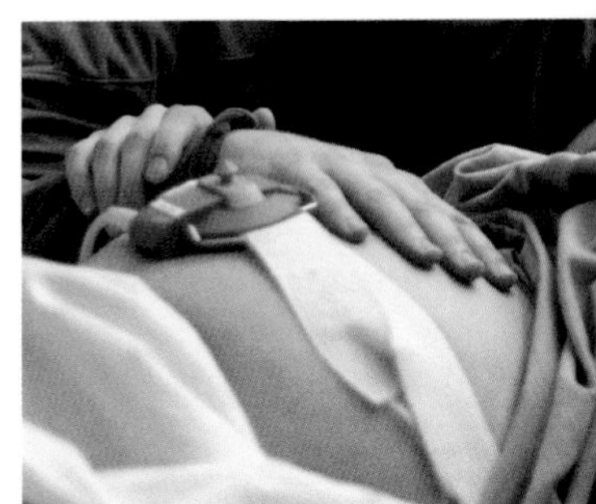

fetus is becoming distressed and may have difficulty tolerating further labor, an emergency C-section may be required.

DID YOU KNOW?

EPIDURAL

An epidural is a regional anesthetic that is commonly used in labor for both normal vaginal deliveries and C-sections. Generally felt to be very safe, it provides a high level of anesthesia to the lower abdomen, with little effect on the heart, lungs, and brain.

An epidural requires the injection of medication into the sac of fluid that surrounds the nerves in the lower end of your spine. The anesthesiologist will carefully clean the area and numb the skin. A needle is then placed into the space between your vertebrae, and a catheter is usually left in place so more medication can be instilled as needed.

Once the epidural is working, your legs and pelvis will feel numb, and you will not be able to control your bladder. When the medication wears off, you will regain complete sensation.

Indications for a Caesarian Section

- The baby's position in the uterus (feet, buttocks, or shoulder first) makes it unlikely that you will be able to safely deliver vaginally.
- There is an anatomical problem. For example, if the placenta is implanted very low in the uterus, the baby's descent could cause massive bleeding.
- There is a high risk that the uterus will rupture because you have undergone previous uterine surgeries.
- You have an underlying medical condition, such as heart disease, active genital herpes, or poorly controlled diabetes.
- There is more than one baby. Twins or triplets may sometimes be delivered by C-section.

Procedure

C-sections are often done while the mother is awake, but with an epidural or spinal anesthetic administered. This means you should feel no pain in the area of the surgery while it is being performed.

The average hospital stay after a C-section varies from 2 to 3 days, although mothers are encouraged to get out of bed as early as possible. Full recovery can take 4 to 6 weeks. Mothers who deliver vaginally usually require only a 1- to 2-day hospital stay, and they make a full recovery more quickly.

Episiotomy

This procedure involves cutting the skin and subcutaneous tissues between the vagina and anus to enlarge the vaginal opening, providing extra space for the baby to emerge through at the time of birth. An episiotomy may also prevent these tissues from tearing. The area will be numbed with a local anesthetic.

Episiotomies are not considered routine and are not always necessary. They do not always prevent the skin from tearing at the time of the birth, although the tear is likely to be smaller and to heal more easily. Speak to your health-care provider about her approach to episiotomies, and discuss the pros and cons ahead of time.

Vacuum or Forceps Delivery

Certain circumstances, such as maternal exhaustion, require assistance with a vacuum or forceps for safe delivery. A vacuum has a suction cup that fits on top of the baby's head. Forceps, which are shaped like steel spoons, can be placed into the vagina, around the baby's head. With each contraction, the mother pushes down and the doctor pulls on the vacuum or forceps to help guide the baby's head out of the vagina. You may see some swelling on the baby's scalp or bruising on his cheeks, but this will disappear over a few days.

Baby's Arrival

Most babies have a vertex presentation, meaning the head is the first part to be delivered. Then it's time for the rest of the body to emerge. The moment you've been waiting for has finally arrived!

DID YOU KNOW?

CUTTING THE CORD

The umbilical cord, which connects the baby to the placenta, is cut using a pair of surgical scissors. This is painless. Cutting the umbilical cord can sometimes be a ceremonial act done by the mother's partner.

Warming Your Baby

After ensuring a clear airway, drying and warming your baby are the first items on the agenda. Cold air is a shock to a newborn, who has spent 9 months surrounded by warm amniotic fluid. Warm blankets are used to dry your baby, and delivery rooms are equipped with a radiant warmer (a small table with overhead heaters) to help keep your baby warm.

If there are no other concerns, your baby can immediately be placed on your abdomen to be warmed with his skin against yours. Once he is warm, dry, and breathing comfortably, he will be weighed, swaddled in a receiving blanket, and given to you or one of your support people to hold.

Apgar Score

More than 90% of newborns make the transition from fetal to extrauterine life smoothly and do not require any further intervention. To aid the health-care team in assessing the baby's ease of adaptation, an Apgar score is assigned at least twice during the baby's first few minutes of life, usually at the first and fifth minutes. The Apgar score, developed in 1952 by Dr. Virginia Apgar, is a numerical score between 0 and 10. It is based on the baby's heart rate, respirations, muscle tone, response to stimulus, and color.

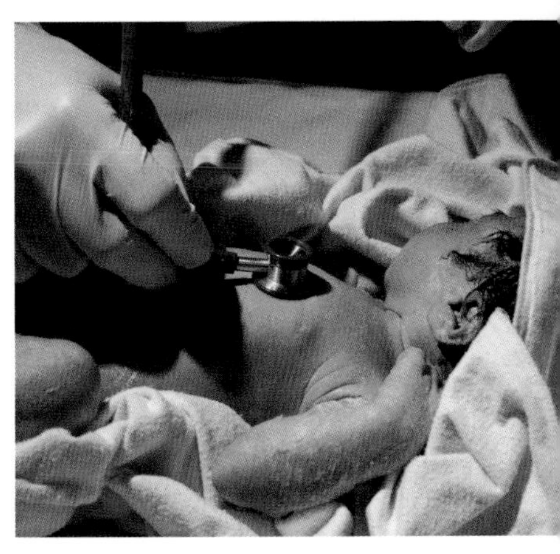

Apgar Score Card

SIGN	SCORE			TOTAL
	0	1	2	
Heart rate	Absent	Slow (<100 bpm)	>100 bpm	
Respirations	Absent	Slow, irregular	Good, crying	
Muscle tone	Limp	Some flexion	Active motion	
Reflex irritability	No response	Grimace	Cough, sneeze, cry	
Color	Blue or pale	Pink body, blue extremities	Completely pink	
				/10

Keep in mind that the score is not a predictor of long-term health. A low score alerts the health-care team that the newborn may need continued medical intervention or simply further observation. A difficult delivery or prematurity are the more common reasons for lower Apgar scores. Even a perfectly healthy baby rarely scores 10 out of 10.

Birthing Features

Most babies are not picture-perfect, at least not immediately, so don't be surprised! Features to be prepared for include the vernix caseosa, which is a white waxy coating covering the baby's skin. Some blood may be on the baby from the delivery process. There may be bruises, and possibly marks from instruments (forceps or vacuum) used during the birth. Acrocyanosis (bluish hands and feet) is both common and normal at this early stage.

Your baby's face may be puffy and slightly misshapen, and the head may be molded as a result of having been delivered through the vaginal canal. Many babies with significant molding have an accompanying caput, a diffuse swelling of the scalp, which heals on its own in just a few days.

Some babies have well-demarcated bumps called cephalohematomas, which are large bruises under the scalp. While they are usually harmless, cephalohematomas usually take a few weeks or even months to heal.

KEY POINT

Regardless of any slight physical imperfections, your baby will be beautiful, and your memories of your baby's birth will undoubtedly be indelible.

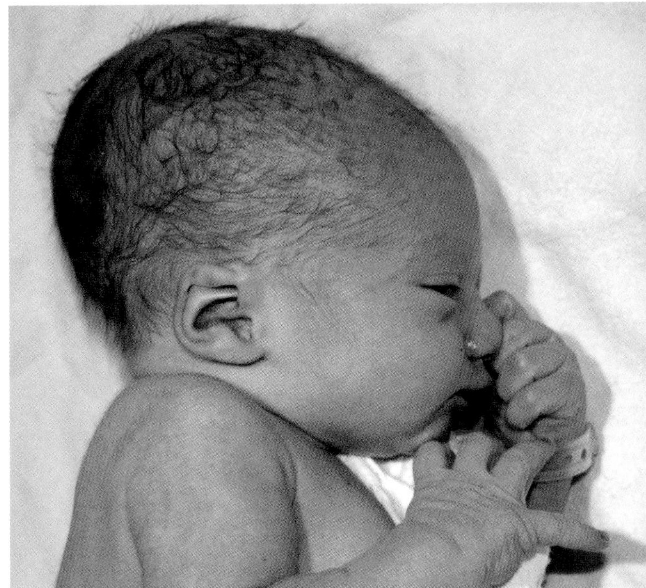

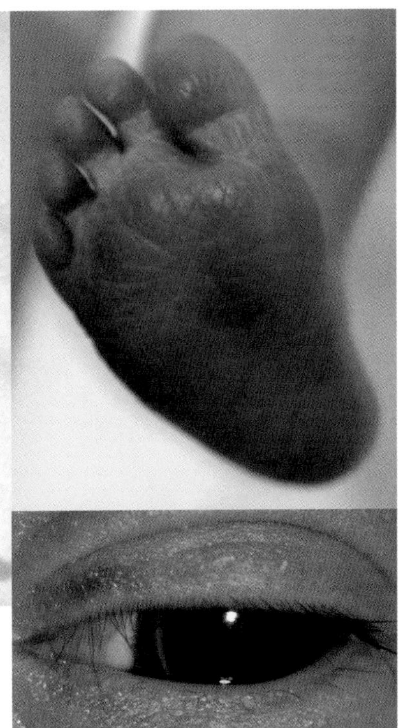

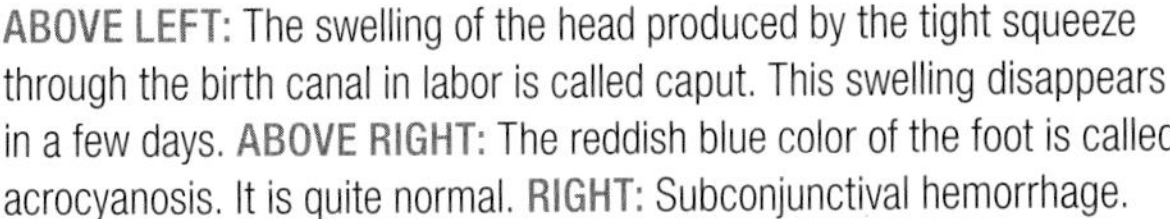

ABOVE LEFT: The swelling of the head produced by the tight squeeze through the birth canal in labor is called caput. This swelling disappears in a few days. **ABOVE RIGHT:** The reddish blue color of the foot is called acrocyanosis. It is quite normal. **RIGHT:** Subconjunctival hemorrhage.

Some babies may also have a subconjunctival hemorrhage. This red streak in the white of the eye results from increased pressure during delivery that causes some bleeding in the vessels of the baby's eye. Subconjunctival hemorrhages are completely harmless. You don't need to worry or do anything special; the blood will disappear on its own within a few days.

Eye Ointment

Antibiotic eye ointment is given to all babies soon after birth to prevent serious eye infections that might occur in the first month.

While most eye infections and discharge are minor, some may be caused by a bacterium (*Neisseria gonorrhea*) that can lead to permanent visual loss. Gonorrhea often causes no symptoms in affected women, but may be contracted by the baby during delivery. The American Academy of Pediatrics and the Canadian Paediatric Society recommend that *all* women be screened for this infection during their pregnancy, and most jurisdictions require every infant to be treated with an eye ointment. This ointment is an antibiotic, generally erythromycin, which is squeezed from a small tube into each eye.

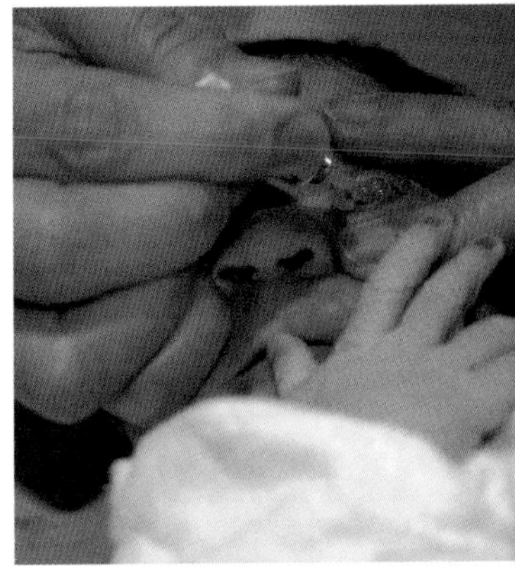

GUIDE TO: Birthmarks

Approximately 20% to 40% of infants have a form of birthmark. Most of these are normal and harmless, and often fade over time, but a small number of birthmarks are signs of an important medical condition.

Salmon Patch (Nevus Simplex)

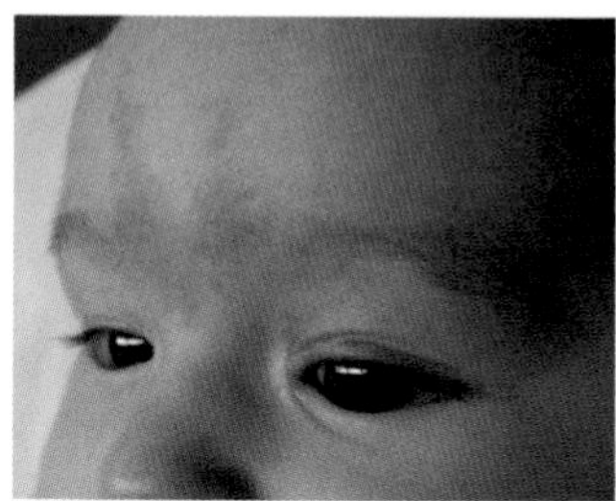

One of the most common birthmarks is the salmon patch — a flat, pink-red area apparent in the newborn period. These typically appear on the eyelid (angel's kiss) or on the back of the neck around the hairline (stork bite). The majority of eyelid marks disappear by themselves over the first year; those on the neck often persist throughout life.

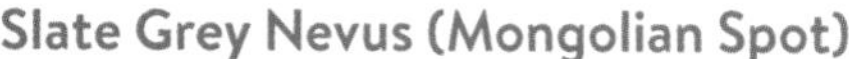

Slate Grey Nevus (Mongolian Spot)

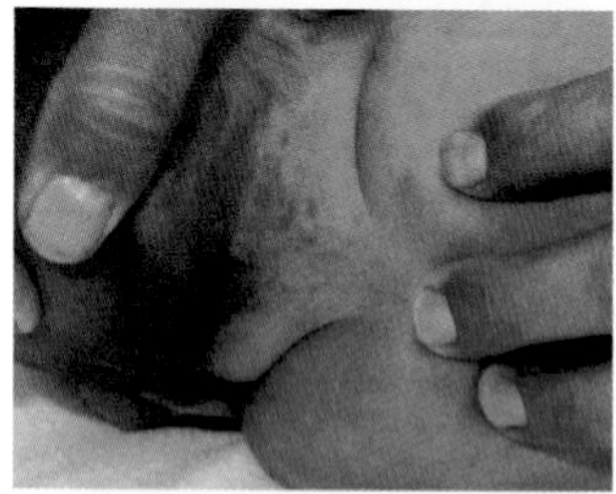

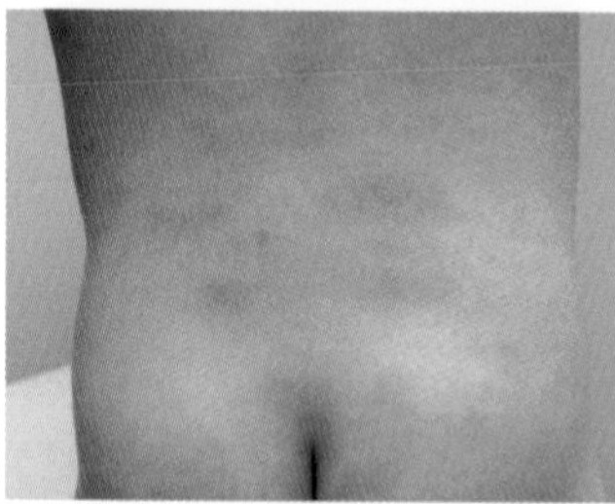

A type of skin pigmentation usually found across the buttocks and lower spine, especially in dark-skinned babies, these spots are flat, bluish-gray in color, and resemble a bruise, except that the color does not change. The markings disappear in 95% of children by the time they reach school age. No treatment is required.

Hemangioma

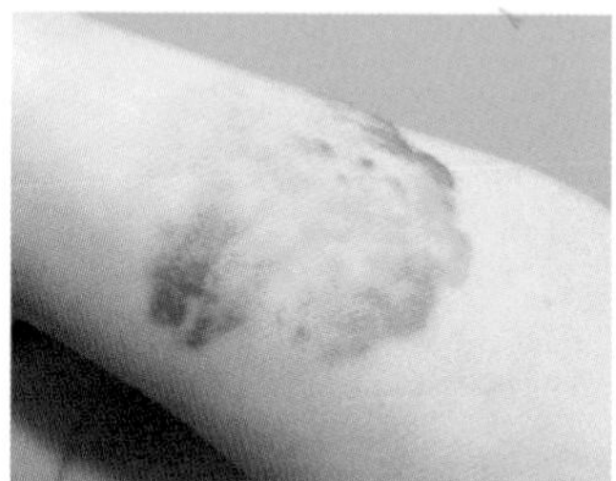

Hemangiomas are growths of immature blood vessels; they can appear as raised, firm, red areas (strawberries) or bluish lumps arising from the deeper skin and tissues. The growths, appearing most often on the face, scalp, and chest, are very common. They are typically very small or absent at birth but have a rapid growth phase (out of proportion to that of the infant) during the first 6 months, then shrink over a period of years. Approximately 60% disappear by age 6 and 90% by age 9. Hemangiomas do not require treatment unless they are in sensitive areas where they may obscure vision or are prone to bleeding.

Port Wine Stain

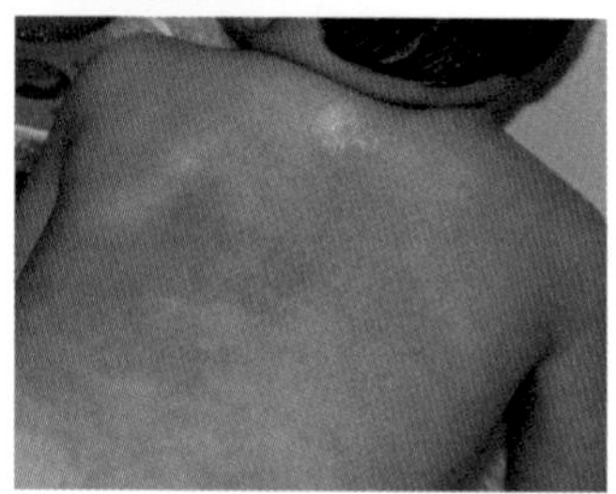

This flat, red-purple mark, made up of mature blood vessels, is evident at birth and grows in proportion to the child. Marks may be treated with laser therapy if they are extensive or in cosmetically important areas.

Vitamin K

Vitamin K is essential for normal blood clotting to occur. It is given to all newborns within the first 6 hours of birth to prevent serious bleeding, a condition called hemorrhagic disease of the newborn. This bleeding can occur unexpectedly, as early as the first day of life and as late as 2 months of age. The most effective way to give vitamin K to the newborn infant is via an injection into the muscle of the baby's upper thigh. This method of administration is the same as the one used later for your baby's early immunizations.

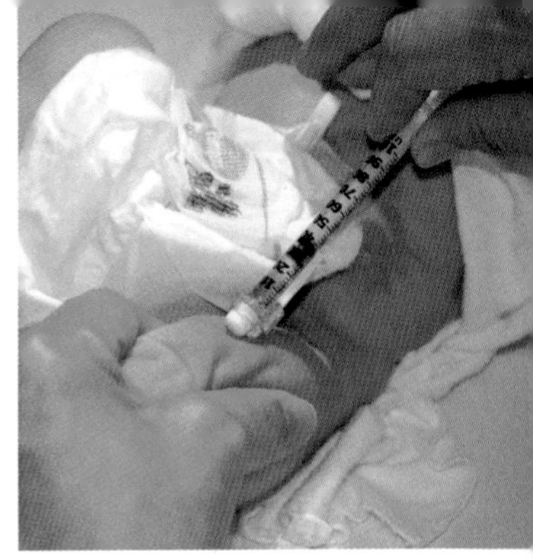

Hospital Stay

Provided that you are both healthy, you and your baby will stay in the same room from birth until hospital discharge. A small bassinet for the baby is usually set up alongside your bed, and the two of you will be cared for by the same nurse.

This is a time for you to begin to get comfortable handling your baby, swaddling him, feeding him, and listening for his cues. You will begin to understand and respond to your baby's needs. If yours has been an uncomplicated delivery, your stay in the hospital may be as brief as 24 to 48 hours. You're certainly not expected to learn all about your baby in that short a time, but it's an important start. Your nurse is there to help, so don't hesitate to ask questions as they arise.

You may not be able to room in with your baby if you are too unwell to care for him or if he requires closer observation or treatment in the nursery. In this situation, your caregivers will make it easy for the two of you to spend as much time together as you both can handle. In many cases, you will have an opportunity to spend at least one night rooming in together before you are discharged.

Baby Checkup

Before you leave the hospital, your newborn will have a complete physical exam by a family doctor, pediatrician, or midwife to ensure he is healthy and ready for discharge. If you already have a doctor picked out for your baby, and your doctor has privileges at the hospital where you are delivering, she will likely come herself to meet and examine her new little patient. Otherwise, the hospital will have the on-call doctor perform the exam; you don't need to worry about making the arrangements.

DID YOU KNOW?

NURSING RIGHT AWAY

If you have chosen to breast-feed your baby, there is no better time to start than right in the delivery room. Most infants are awake and ready to learn how to nurse in the first 2 hours of life. Provided that your baby has adapted to life outside the womb and is stable, he can be placed on your abdomen, skin to skin, within minutes of birth. Many babies in this position, when given time, will find the breast on their own, latch on, and begin to feed. Even if the baby doesn't feed right away, the skin-to-skin contact itself has been shown to be good for the newborn: it keeps him warm and stabilizes vital parameters, such as heart rate and breathing.

Size

Your doctor will note your baby's weight and measure his length and head circumference. She will plot these measurements on a graph that shows how big your baby is in comparison to other newborns. How your baby compares with others is not in itself important, but rather provides a reference point from which your child's growth can be followed over time. You should make a note of these initial measurements and keep a record of them.

Head to Toe

Your doctor will observe your baby to evaluate his general appearance, listen to his chest with a stethoscope, feel his head, neck, hips, and belly, and check his newborn reflexes. However, much of the exam is done by simply observing how your baby looks and behaves while being examined.

DID YOU KNOW?

TESTING PROTOCOLS

There is considerable variation regarding testing protocols for newborn screening. Some jurisdictions are now employing techniques to test for many disorders with just one small blood sample. These conditions are individually quite uncommon, but, cumulatively, they add up to a lot of babies whose lives can be improved by early detection and treatment. Across most jurisdictions in North America, babies are typically tested for at least three conditions: phenylketonuria (PKU), congenital hypothyroidism, and hearing disorders.

Blood Tests

Many disorders are, unfortunately, not apparent at birth, even with a complete newborn physical exam. Though most of these conditions are rare, significant strides have been made in managing them if they are detected in a timely manner. With this in mind, all babies born in developed countries are screened for certain conditions.

Most of these diseases are related to a problem with genetics, metabolism, blood, or hormones. They can be tested with a blood sample. Your nurse or midwife will take the sample by pricking your baby's heel, then squeezing out a few drops of blood onto special paper.

Most tests are accurate only if the blood sample is taken after the baby is 24 hours old. If you and your baby are discharged from the hospital before this time, make sure that arrangements are made to have your doctor or midwife do the testing at the appropriate time. The results often take more than a week or two and will be sent to your doctor, who will notify you if there are any concerns.

Hearing

Simple non-invasive methods are available to test a newborn baby's hearing. Hearing loss is one of the most common congenital conditions, affecting approximately three in 1,000 babies. Up to half of all babies with hearing loss have no known risk factors that will alert caregivers to an increased probability of hearing deficit. It is vital to detect hearing loss before 6 months of age because intervening from this early stage markedly improves the chances that the baby's speech and language will develop normally. This makes screening all babies particularly important. Most communities in the United States and Canada offer universal screening before you leave the hospital.

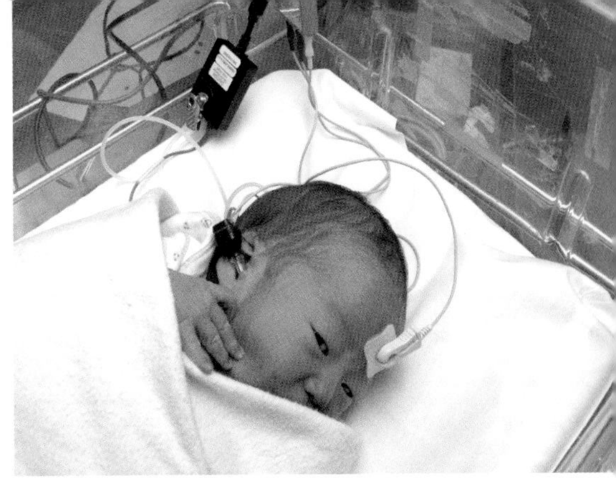

Newborn screening for hearing loss.

Jaundice

Your baby's routine assessments in the first days of life will include monitoring for the yellow color that indicates jaundice and checking for signs of hydration, as well as tracking your baby's weight to monitor how well the initiation of feeding is going. While jaundice is easiest to see in Caucasian babies, it is evident in darker-skinned babies by looking at the whites of their eyes, the palms of their hands and the soles of their feet.

KEY POINT

If your baby is healthy, and the bilirubin level is not too high, the jaundice is harmless and will resolve naturally.

Jaundice Facts

Jaundice is caused by excess bilirubin — a product of the natural breakdown of red blood cells. Normally, bilirubin is processed through the liver and excreted primarily in the stool. In newborn babies, several aspects of bilirubin metabolism are not yet fully developed, resulting in the common appearance of jaundice.

Jaundice typically begins in a full-term infant after the first 24 hours of life. The bilirubin level peaks at 3 to 5 days, and then gradually decreases over approximately 2 to 3 weeks. Since bilirubin is excreted in the stool, an important component of clearing jaundice is to ensure that babies are well hydrated and passing meconium stools (see page 40), which is generally accomplished by establishing feeds.

Jaundice begins by affecting the whites of the baby's eyes; as the bilirubin level increases, the yellow appears to spread downward, from head to toe.

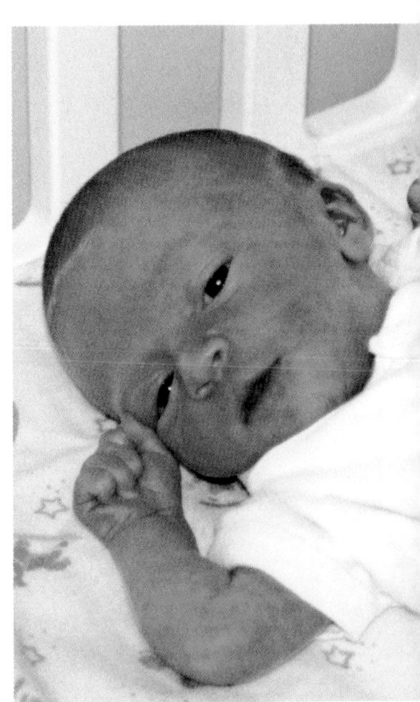

Testing for Jaundice

Most babies will be screened for jaundice in the first few days of life. This is usually done by taking a blood sample — usually by means of a simple heel prick. While most jaundice is harmless, very high bilirubin levels can affect the brain, a consequence avoided by monitoring and treatment. The majority of babies whose bilirubin levels are a bit high only require that levels are checked until the doctor is confident that the jaundice is decreasing. Graphs advise health-care providers of when treatment of jaundice is necessary based on the age of the newborn and various other factors.

DID YOU KNOW?

WEIGHT LOSS

Newborns may lose up to 10% of their birth weight over the first few days of life due to the loss of fluids and the elimination of meconium after birth. Babies also have minimal intake initially, particularly if they are breast-feeding. A small amount of weight loss (less than 10% of birth weight) may be acceptable. However, your baby's weight should be followed closely at the beginning to ensure that he does not lose too much and that he begins to appropriately gain it back, both signs that he is getting enough milk and is not dehydrated. He should regain his birth weight by 10 to 14 days of age, and then will gain about ⅔ to 1 ounce (20 to 30 g) per day over the first 3 months.

▷ Jaundice Red Flags

There are several reasons why jaundice might persist, or be thought to be significant. Prematurity is one of the more common ones, as is blood group incompatibility (where a baby inherits his blood group from his father, and his mother carries antibodies that break down some of his red blood cells while he is in the womb). In general, there are a few red flags that would indicate that your baby's jaundice is more than just routine:

- His jaundice is apparent within 24 hours of birth.
- He is not feeding well.
- He is not voiding.
- He is not passing meconium.
- He has a fever.
- He is lethargic.

Treatments for Jaundice

Some babies require special ultraviolet lights, a treatment called phototherapy, to help bring the jaundice level down. If phototherapy is needed, your baby will be placed in an incubator with lights surrounding it, with his eyes covered for protection. Although this requires hospitalization, it is a very effective therapy that is harmless and commonly used. Given that hydration is an important part of clearing bilirubin from the body, your baby may require additional fluids if his feeding is not yet established. These fluids may be in the form of supplementation with milk by various methods (cup, syringe, lactation device).

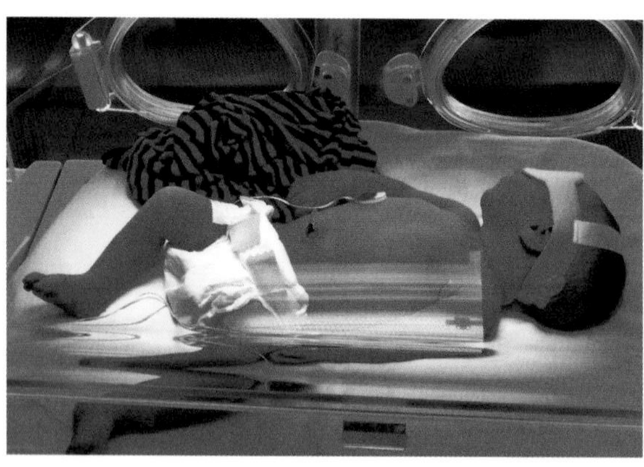

Phototherapy

Common Rashes

Several types of rashes may affect your baby's skin as early as the first day of life. Most are harmless and resolve on their own. There are three common rashes: milia, baby acne and erythema toxicum.

- **Milia:** Milia are tiny white bumps on the skin, most prominent over the bridge of the nose and the cheeks. They are small sebaceous glands containing a buildup of natural oils. They require no treatment and will disappear within a few weeks.
- **Baby acne:** Your baby may get pimples long before puberty hits! Just wash the skin normally and pat dry. The acne will resolve within a few months and should not leave any lasting marks.
- **Erythema toxicum:** This extremely common rash, often noted in the first couple of days of life, consists of a red flat base with a tiny white or yellow pustule in the center. You may see just a few such markings or several over your baby's body. They seem to come and go in different areas, almost before your eyes. This rash is harmless and no treatment is required.

DID YOU KNOW?

LIP BLISTERS

Another common occurrence in the first few weeks of a newborn's life is the formation of a blister, or callus, in the middle of the upper lip. This is due to the baby's vigorous sucking and is completely harmless. There's no need to try to stop your baby from sucking to deal with the blister; sucking is a natural reflex in babies, and the blister will heal on its own.

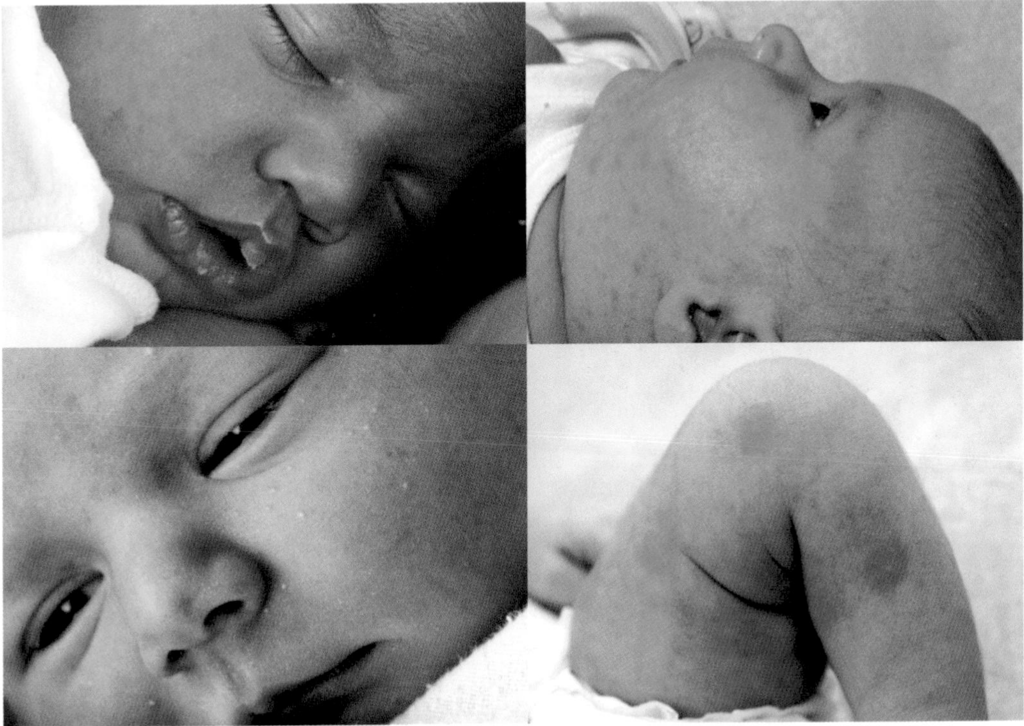

TOP LEFT: Lip blister. **TOP RIGHT:** Baby acne. **Bottom LEFT:** Milia. **BOTTOM RIGHT:** Erythema toxicum

Breast-Feeding Anxiety

While breast-feeding is natural, it is also a learned skill, one that you and your baby will become expert at over time. Remembering that both of you will learn with experience helps to alleviate the anxiety that many mothers feel. The most important initial step is to ensure that your baby has a proper latch (see page 61). This will help to avoid sore or cracked nipples and will optimize your baby's milk intake. With this in mind, don't hesitate to ask for help. Nurses, midwives, and lactation consultants are all valuable resources.

DID YOU KNOW?

LACTATION CONSULTANTS

Breast-feeding can be a rewarding but challenging task, especially in the very beginning. Check with your public health department to see if they offer breast-feeding help, or access a lactation consultant by contacting either your birth hospital or La Leche League (a breast-feeding support group).

Quality, Not Quantity

Nursing at this early stage is not about quantity. Healthy full-term babies do not need to be fed immediately. When they do begin to nurse, they will benefit from colostrum, the special breast milk that is produced before regular breast milk comes in. Colostrum is high in immunoglobulins — proteins that will strengthen your baby's immune system — and while it is not produced in large quantities, it is all your baby needs for the first few days.

DID YOU KNOW?

INFECTION RISK

Whether in the hospital or at home, keep in mind that, like all newborns, yours will be vulnerable to infection. Anybody who is ill should stay away until fully recovered; if visitors do not display this common courtesy, don't hesitate to politely ask them to delay their visit until they are no longer sick. All guests should wash their hands before holding the baby. Toddlers who visit should be supervised and guided to gently touch the baby if they wish (after hand-washing), but should avoid touching his face and hands.

Be Flexible

There are sometimes circumstances in which the baby requires medical attention and is not able to nurse right away. Rest assured that your baby's caregivers have his best interests at heart. The nursery staff will assist you with expressing milk and preparing you for the time when breast-feeding becomes possible. Remember that many babies who are not nursed right away are still successfully breast-fed.

Leaving the Hospital

Upon hospital discharge, many parents feel as though they are being "let loose" with a new baby to care for — and no idea where to begin. What will hopefully be one of the most wonderful periods of your life will also, undoubtedly, be physically and emotionally challenging. Every new parent requires support, so don't be afraid to accept offers or ask for help.

Don't forget to take care of yourself as well! You will have a scheduled postpartum visit with your obstetrician, family doctor, or midwife, but don't hesitate to make additional visits if you have questions or concerns about your own physical or emotional health. Friends, relatives, and your public health department can all be of assistance.

Newborns' Sleep Patterns

Countless hours lie ahead when you will interact with your wakeful new baby; just don't expect this to start immediately. Nature seems to have told our little ones that mothers need rest following labor and delivery.

In the first day or two of life, babies are usually very quiet and sleepy. They have some recovering of their own to do! By the second night, newborns are often much more awake, and you will more than likely hear their frequent cry. Over the first few weeks, babies generally sleep for periods of 2 to 4 hours, wake with a cry, feed, and settle back to sleep. Babies often even doze off during a feed. A diaper change midway through, or between sides if you're nursing, will help to stimulate the baby and allow him to finish his meal. Though a newborn's alert periods are initially very brief, they will gradually lengthen, and by a month of age, babies are usually alert for a few hours a day.

Keep in mind that there is considerable individual variation in these patterns; as long as your baby is thriving, there is no "right" or "wrong" amount of time for him to be awake or asleep.

Evening Routine

Some babies differentiate day from night faster than others, sleeping longer stretches at night. As long as your baby is growing well, there is usually no need to wake him for feedings. As your baby gets older, to encourage him to recognize when it's nighttime, try to initiate an evening routine early on: a warm bath, reading a story, or listening to or singing the same lullaby each night.

REM Sleep

During longer stretches of sleep, you may hear your baby murmuring or stirring. He is likely in the REM (rapid eye movement) stage of sleep, which is naturally accompanied by movement. If you pick him up in response to every little sound, you may actually be disturbing the natural rhythm of sleep. If he seems comfortable but is simply stirring or making gentle sounds, let him be until he truly cries, indicating that his sleep cycle is over.

DID YOU KNOW?

SLEEP WHEN YOUR BABY SLEEPS

Whatever your baby's pattern, you should try your best to sleep when the baby is sleeping. This is a period when mothers are recovering from the birthing process, learning how to breast-feed, and adjusting to their baby's round-the-clock feeding schedule. Few new parents are well rested, but making an effort to sleep when you can will help to keep your body healthy and your mind clear, allowing you to take better care of your newborn.

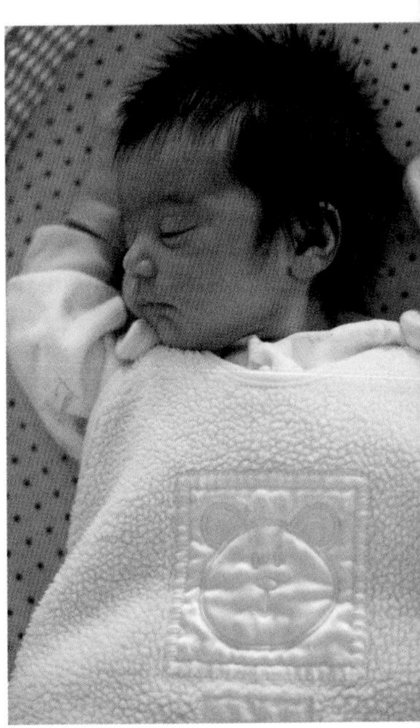

That said, when your baby does cry, it's important to respond. For at least the first 4 to 6 months, it is important to foster a sense of security. You can accomplish this in part by responding to your baby's cues, teaching him that you are there for him when he needs you.

For more information on helping your baby sleep, see Chapter 5, page 110.

HOW TO: Swaddle Your Baby

Many babies find comfort in being tightly bundled, perhaps feeling closer to their 9 months spent warm and snug in the womb. You can learn how to swaddle your baby from the nurse or midwife caring for you and your baby after the delivery, but the basic approach is as follows:

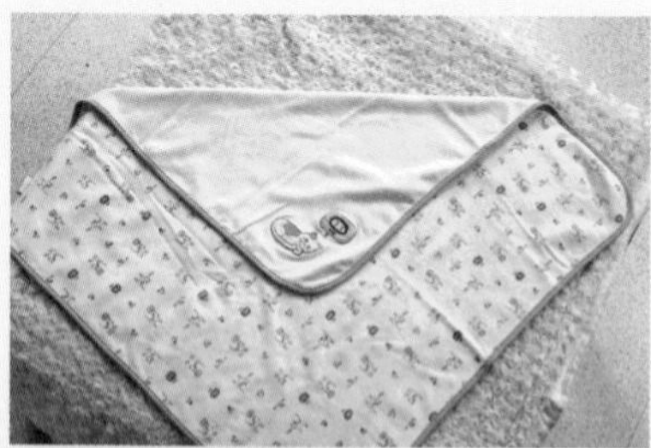

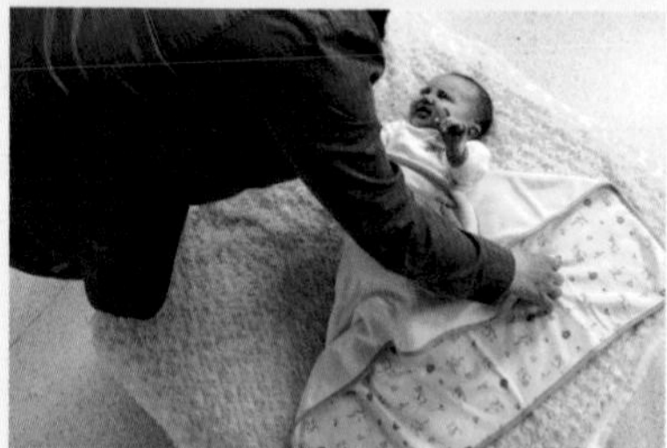

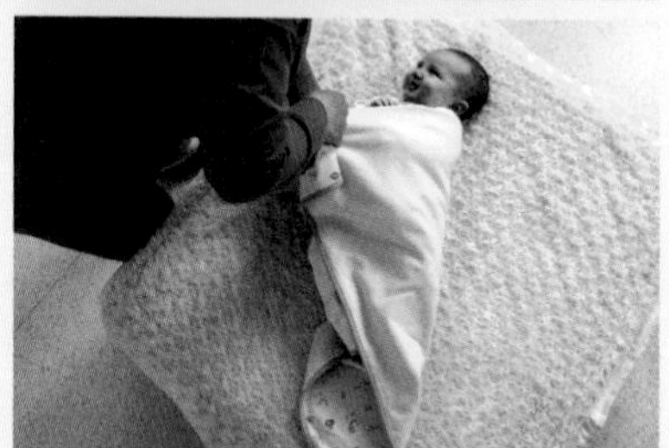

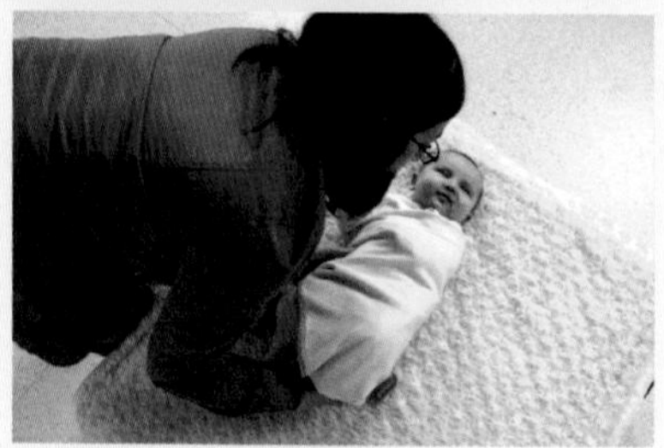

1. Use a large, square receiving blanket, if possible.
2. Lay it in front of you like a diamond and fold the top corner down to the blanket's center.
3. Lay your baby on his back with his head just above the folded corner.
4. Holding his right arm down alongside his body, bring the left side of the blanket over his shoulder and down across his body, tucking it snugly under the left side of his body.
5. Bring the top of the right side of the blanket down just a little, to cover the left shoulder, and wrap the remaining blanket across your baby's body, tucking it under him on the right.
6. Straighten his left arm along his side while you bring the bottom corner up, tucking the blanket under his left shoulder and around his side.
7. Make the wrap fairly snug – loose blankets are unsafe for little babies.
8. If your baby enjoys being swaddled but prefers his hands free, or if you rely on his hand and mouth cues for hunger, you can still follow the technique above, but simply bend your baby's arms at the elbows, leaving his hands free.

Pacifiers

Using a pacifier is a controversial practice. Parents will need to assess the pros and cons based on the needs of their own child.

What are the advantages? A pacifier can be used to satisfy a baby's need to suck in between feedings, which may provide comfort and help him to settle. A pacifier is better than a thumb because it is less likely to cause problems with future tooth development and is easier for the parent to control. Some medical research suggests that using a pacifier may decrease the risk of SIDS (sudden infant death syndrome, or crib death).

What about the disadvantages? Not using a pacifier properly (starting too early or using it for too many hours of the day or for too long) can lead to problems with breast-feeding, dental cavities, overbite, and, possibly, ear infections.

KEY POINT

If you choose to use a pacifier, limit the time you allow your child to suck on it. Allow it at sleep time and to give comfort until 12 months, then plan to give it up.

GUIDE TO: Pacifier Use

- Don't start using one until breast-feeding is established.
- See if your baby is hungry, tired, or bored before resorting to the pacifier.
- Sterilize it in boiling water before first use.
- Don't dip it in sugar or honey.
- Don't tie it around the baby's neck (this can cause strangulation); instead, use a clip with a short thread.
- Don't use it all day long.

Urine and Stool Patterns

After having a baby, you will probably discuss voiding patterns and bowel movements much more than you ever thought possible! A newborn's voiding and stooling patterns are, in fact, very important because they indicate whether he is getting enough to eat. This is particularly true in breast-fed infants, because the quantity of their intake is difficult to assess.

Urine

If you're breast-feeding, don't expect your baby's diapers to be soaking wet until your milk comes in, usually after

2 to 5 days. Remember that, at first, your baby will be getting colostrum, the initial form of breast milk. Generally speaking, colostrum is about quality rather than quantity, so don't fret too much about the volume produced.

It can often be difficult to estimate urine production. Absorbent disposable diapers make judging whether your baby has voided, and how much, particularly difficult. So can the mixing of urine with soft stools. Other indicators, such as weight and a physical assessment of hydration by your health-care provider, can serve as indirect signs that your baby is adequately hydrated.

Stools

Your baby's first bowel movements, formed in the intestines before birth, will be black and sticky. This excrement, called meconium, should be eliminated over the first 2 to 3 days of life. If it persists beyond that, it may be a sign that feeding is not progressing appropriately and that your baby is at increased risk for dehydration and jaundice, something you should check with his doctor.

Following the meconium, stools will gradually transition from brown to green to yellow. Breast-fed babies have very loose and seedy bowel movements, whereas the stools of bottle-fed babies tend to be more pasty yellow.

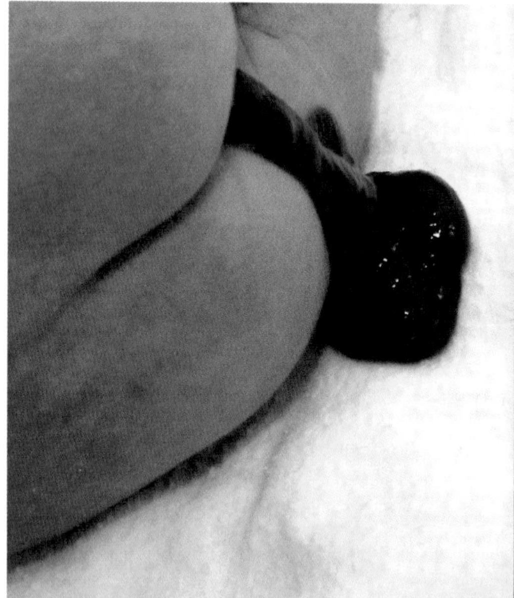

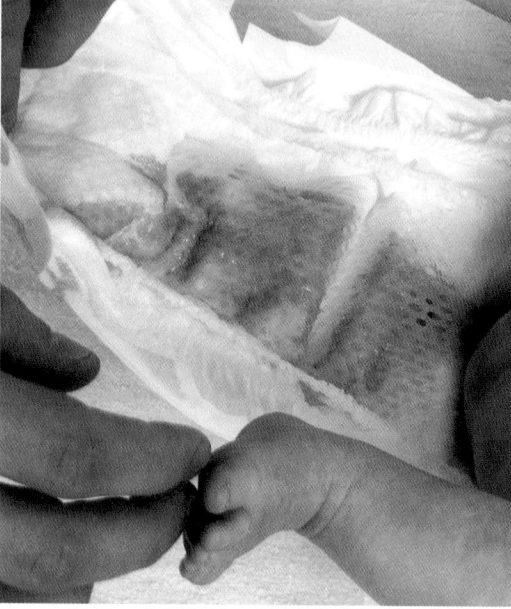

Your baby's first bowel movement will appear black and sticky. This stool is called meconium. Once your breast milk comes in, the stools will become a yellowish color with a soft and seedy consistency.

Newborn Urine and Stool Patterns

BABY'S AGE	WET DIAPERS EACH DAY	STOOLS EACH DAY
1 day old	At least 1 wet diaper	At least 1 to 2 sticky dark green/black stools
2 days old	At least 2 wet diapers	At least 1 to 2 sticky dark green/black stools
3 days old	At least 3 heavy wet diapers	At least 2 to 3 brown/green/yellow stools
4 days old	At least 4 heavy wet diapers	At least 2 to 3 brown/green/yellow stools
5 days old	At least 5 heavy wet diapers	At least 2 to 3 stools getting more yellow
6 days old and after	At least 6 heavy wet diapers. At all ages, urine should be clear to pale yellow with almost no smell.	At least 2 to 3 large yellow stools. Stools can be soft like toothpaste or seedy and watery.

Changing Diapers

Of all the joys that accompany having a baby, endless diaper changes are probably not high on your list! However, they are a necessary part of parenthood and will become a part of your routine.

There are no rules about how often to change a baby's diaper. Clearly, if he has had a bowel movement or is uncomfortable, it's time for a diaper change. Otherwise, a good routine in the newborn period is to change the diaper either before or after a feed. You might find that changing your baby at the start of a feed is a good tactic, not only to ensure a clean diaper, but to stimulate him so he is alert for his feeding.

KEY POINT

There is no need to wake a sleeping baby just to change his diaper.

Equipment

Newborn Diapers

A supply of clean diapers is, of course, essential! Though you'll need to buy some diapers before your baby is born, don't stock up on too many in the newborn size. Even average-size babies will quickly outgrow them, and it's better for diapers to fit slightly big than too small.

HOW TO: Change a Diaper

1. With your clean diaper and wipes ready to go, place your baby on his back and undo his current diaper by undoing the tapes at either side. (If you're using cloth diapers, there are systems available with Velcro tabs.)
2. If there's a bowel movement, use the dirty diaper to wipe away some of the stool as you pull the diaper out from under the baby. Roll the dirty diaper up and secure it with the tapes or tabs.
3. Lifting your baby's legs by the ankles, wipe him clean with a baby wipe or wet cotton pad, being sure to get into the creases. For girls, remember to wipe from front to back.
4. Slip a clean, open diaper under your baby, with the tapes or tabs at the back.
5. Bring the front of the diaper up between his legs, open the tapes or tabs, and fasten them snugly on either side. Until the umbilical stump has fallen off, fold the top edge of the diaper down below the cord to prevent irritation.
6. For boys, ensure that the penis is aimed down when securing the clean diaper to minimize leakage out the top. Also, try to keep the penis covered with a clean diaper during the change to protect everybody in the vicinity!
7. Always wash your hands after a diaper change. If it is difficult to get to the sink with baby in tow, keep a bottle of alcohol-based hand sanitizer by the change table.

Count on using about 80 diapers per week for the first month of your baby's life. Once you're sure that he will be in one size for a while, check out discount stores or bulk sections, where disposable diapers will often be boxed in larger quantities at much lower prices.

DID YOU KNOW?

CHANGE OF CLOTHES

Despite proper diapering technique, babies often soil or wet not just their diaper but their clothes too, so make sure to have a change of clothes or an extra sleeper available!

Baby Wipes

You will also need baby wipes to wipe the baby's diaper area after a bowel movement. For sensitive newborn skin, either use a hypoallergenic, fragrance-free commercial brand or buy a supply of cotton pads or towelettes, which can be wet with warm water. The latter are often available at medical or surgical supply stores, and a small spray bottle of water kept by the change table will make wetting them convenient, eliminating a last-minute dash to the closest sink.

Skin Creams

A petroleum jelly, such as Vaseline, may be useful for minor irritations or keeping dry skin moist. A zinc-based barrier cream will cure many diaper rashes by providing a barrier between the baby's stool and his skin. If a rash is not responding to these simple solutions, have your doctor take a look. A mild steroid cream may be prescribed to reduce the inflammation. A simple yeast infection, which is easily treated, may be diagnosed.

If your baby's diaper area is clear, clean, and dry, no ointment or cream is necessary.

Bathing Your Baby

Newborn babies are small, squirmy, and slippery. It's no wonder that the thought of bathing one is enough to make a new parent's heart race! Relax. Before you know it, giving your baby a bath will be just one of many new tasks at which you are an expert. Your nurse will give your baby his first bath before he leaves the hospital. This is a wonderful opportunity for you to watch, learn, and ask questions.

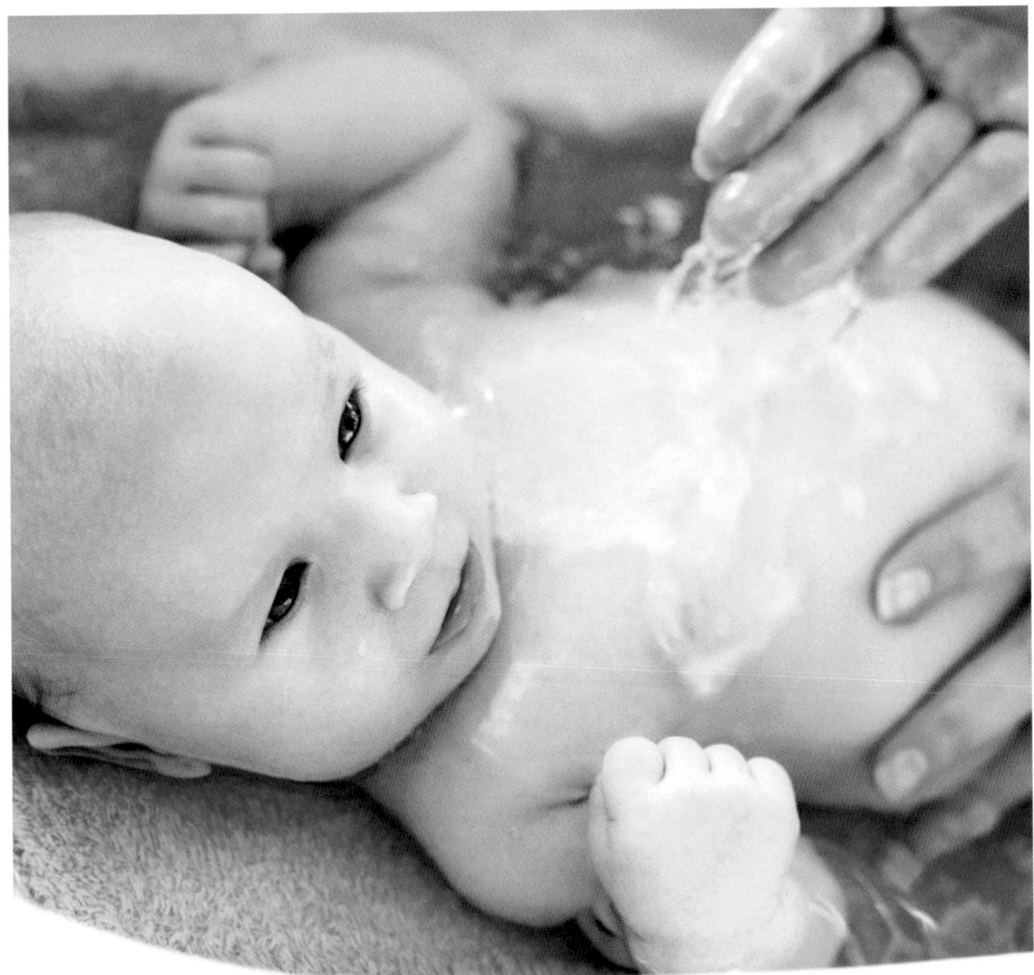

Bathing Routine

You do not need to bathe your baby every day. Before he begins to crawl and get really dirty, two to three times a week is adequate. Of course, the diaper area should be cleaned well with each diaper change, and, if your baby tends to spit up, it is helpful to use a damp washcloth to clean the baby's neck folds.

With time, you may find that your baby's baths have become a part of his routine, enjoyed by you both. In this case, feel free to bathe your baby as often as you like. However, if your baby's skin is sensitive, try limiting the use of baby wash to two to three times per week. The rest of the time, simply bathe with water.

> **DID YOU KNOW?**
>
> **BATHING SCHEDULE**
>
> There is no right or wrong time of the day to give your baby a bath, though many parents find that the warm water helps to relax their baby before bedtime and helps to establish a bedtime routine. Try to avoid a bath time when your baby is likely to be hungry, because he will inevitably be upset. It is also not a good idea to bathe a small infant immediately after a feed because he is more likely to spit up.

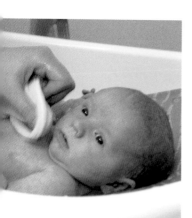

Equipment

Have the following items prepared before you undress your baby, to minimize the time that he is undressed and exposed to the cold.

- Baby wash (milder than soap; avoid dyes and perfumes)
- Washcloth
- Towel (a hooded one is not essential but is nice to have)
- Clean diaper
- Fresh clothing or sleepers

Sponge Baths vs. Full Baths

You may wash your baby by giving either a sponge bath or a full bath. Both are fine right from the beginning.

Sponge Baths

1. Choose a stable surface to set the baby down on, such as a change table, counter, or bed.
2. Cover the surface with a waterproof pad or towel.
3. Make sure your water supply — either a sink or a basin filled with warm water — is close enough that you can keep at least one hand on the baby the entire time.
4. In the newborn period, you may be more comfortable holding your baby in your arms while you give him a sponge bath rather than setting him down.
5. Put some baby wash on a damp washcloth, soap up one area at a time, rinse with clean water, and pat dry.
6. While there is no magic order in which to wash your baby's body, the general rule is to wash from "clean to

dirty," so you don't contaminate the cleanest areas of the body.

7. Wash your baby's eyes by gently wiping the washcloth across the closed eye.
8. Wash girls' genitalia from front to back.
9. Remember to wash your baby's fingers and toes and to dry well in between each digit.

Full Baths

1. You can bathe your baby directly in the sink or use a small portable tub. Given the need to fully support the baby at this early stage, the sink is often easiest because it puts the baby at a comfortable level.
2. Ensure that the sink is well cleaned and its bottom is covered with a rubber mat to prevent the baby from slipping.
3. Fill the bath with warm water — a few inches or centimeters is all that is needed.
4. Undress your baby and gradually slip him into the water.
5. Wash him using the same principles as for sponge baths, soaping up and rinsing the whole body.
6. Pay particular attention to holding your baby's head steady until he gains more neck control.
7. To wash his buttocks and back, turn him over so his tummy rests on your arm.

Safety Tips for Bathing

Although there are very few "rights" or "wrongs" in caring for your baby, there are some safety rules that must be followed when giving him a bath.

1. Always test the water temperature with a sensitive part of your body — your elbow or the underside of your wrist. The water should be warm to the touch, but not hot.
2. Never run the water directly from the tap while your baby is in the bath; unexpected temperature changes may occur.
3. Never leave your baby alone in the bath, even for a second. Babies can drown quickly in even an inch (2.5 cm) of water.
4. Always empty the water immediately after the bath is finished.

DID YOU KNOW?

EAR CARE

Your baby's ears require very little specific attention. The outer ear can be cleaned along with the rest of the body during the baby's bath. There is no reason to stick any object, be it your finger or a Q-tip, into your baby's ear canal. In fact, this is a dangerous practice.

You will see earwax in your baby's ear: it's natural and is the body's way of protecting the eardrum. It does not need to be washed out, but will make its own way to the outside of the ear and fall out. If you're worried that your baby's earwax is blocking his ear, speak to your doctor about your concern rather than attempting to remedy the problem yourself.

GUIDE TO: Penis Care

The penis is made up of the shaft and the rounded end, called the glans, which is covered by the foreskin. Some parents choose to have their son circumcised, others choose not to.

Uncircumcised

At birth, the foreskin is attached to the glans. The two will gradually separate naturally, usually within 2 years, but sometimes over a longer period of time. Do not try to separate the foreskin from the glans; this could be harmful to your baby. At this age, pulling the foreskin back to expose the glans will probably cause more problems than it prevents. Rather, simply wash the penis externally during your baby's bath, using soap and water just as you would the rest of his body.

Circumcised

If you choose to have your baby circumcised, the penis will require some attention for a few days following the procedure. The health-care provider who performs the circumcision will provide you with specific instructions for care. Generally, petroleum jelly is all that is needed. It is applied directly to the penis with every diaper change until the wound is healed. A small amount of bleeding is normal within the first day or two and is not usually a cause for concern. If there is a large amount of blood or the bleeding is not stopping, see your baby's doctor.

Caring for the Umbilical Cord

Immediately following your baby's delivery, a plastic clamp will be placed on the umbilical cord and the cord will be cut. The residual stump is initially white and fleshy, and the three blood vessels through which blood has flowed for the past 9 months are sometimes visible. The plastic clamp will probably be removed before you leave the hospital, and, gradually, the stump will shrivel, dry, and fall off, resulting in the baby's "belly button." The time that the umbilical stump takes to fall off can vary, but it usually occurs within the first 2 weeks after birth. Until that happens, most new parents wonder how to care for the cord.

Studies show that measures such as cleaning the cord with antiseptics or protecting it with gauze dressings offer no advantage over simply keeping it clean and dry. Sponge baths have historically been recommended until the cord separates, but again, there is no evidence that this is a better practice than giving your baby a total body wash and patting the stump dry afterwards.

DID YOU KNOW?

BLOOD STAINS

Don't worry if there is a drop or two of blood on the diaper in the first day or two after the cord falls off: that's normal. You should only be concerned about a steady or persistent oozing of blood.

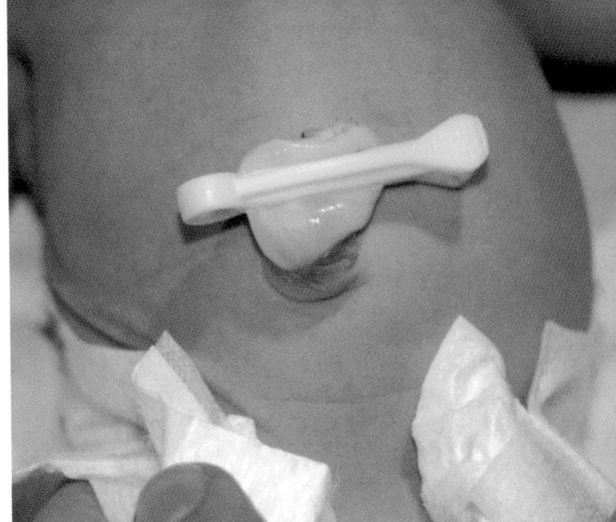

So, what should you do? As with most parts of a healthy baby's body, you don't need to do much!

1. Wash the cord with baby wash and water as part of your newborn's bath and keep it dry between baths.
2. To prevent irritation, fold down the top of the diaper so that it is not rubbing against the cord.
3. Be mindful of signs of infection: warmth, redness, or swelling in the skin immediately surrounding the stump or the presence of pus or other foul-smelling discharge. If any of these arise, contact your baby's doctor immediately.
4. Do not try to hasten the umbilical stump's separation. This will happen naturally.

Dressing Your Baby

Knowing what baby clothes are practical to buy, what your baby will be comfortable wearing, and how to fit your squirmy munchkin into those little clothes can be tricky! Here are some handy guidelines.

1. First, remember that your baby's initial couple of months will consist largely of feeding, sleeping, and being held. From a clothing standpoint, this translates to one thing — sleepers! They are comfortable for the baby whether he is awake or asleep, can be layered with an undershirt or "onesie" (short- or long-sleeved) underneath depending on the season, and snap open at the crotch to make for easy diaper changes.
2. If you buy one-piece sleepers with feet, you won't need to worry about socks, which are always falling off their little feet. Of course, it is fun to take your baby out of a sleeper and dress him in a little outfit once in a while. You'll find that you do this occasionally at first, and increasingly as your baby emerges from the newborn period, until you're in a routine of dressing him in regular clothes during the day, with sleepers reserved for nighttime wear. With this in mind, and remembering that babies grow fast, don't stock up on too many clothes in the 0–3 months size.

DID YOU KNOW?

GIFTS

You might receive many baby clothes as gifts, undoubtedly all well-intentioned and given with love. While you may want to keep some, leave the tags on the clothes until you have time to sort through them. That way, you can make note of duplicates, unnecessary items, or clothing for the wrong season. Many gifts come with gift receipts that make returns easy, but even without a receipt, many stores will accept returns for credit. As your baby grows, you'll have lots of opportunity to buy him new clothes — and the credit note will be much appreciated.

3. Look for items that are easy to put on and take off. With tops or sleepers that have snaps all the way up, you won't have to pull clothing over your baby's head — something no baby enjoys. If you do buy items that pull over his head, make sure there are snaps at the shoulder or overlays of material on either side of the neck designed to stretch easily. Pants or overalls with snaps at the crotch make diaper changes possible without pulling your baby's pants off and on again — a struggle with kicking feet!
4. To keep your baby warm but not overheated, a simple rule of thumb is to dress him as you would dress yourself, adding one thin layer in colder weather. Babies' heads are a major source of heat loss, so it's a good idea to use a cotton hat, even indoors, in colder weather, especially when your baby is sleeping. If you live in a colder climate, appropriate outdoor gear, such as a snowsuit or bunting bag, mittens, and a warm hat, is essential. One-piece snowsuits that zip the entire length will make your life considerably easier. Remember that scarves are a strangling hazard; avoid them for babies and small children.
5. Try reaching up through the sleeve to retrieve your baby's hand and assist it through, rather than struggling to get it through from the top end.
6. For clothing that fits over the head, first stretch the neck of the shirt in your hands, then place either the front under the baby's chin or the back at the back of his head and lift the shirt up. This method will prevent the baby from feeling trapped or smothered by the clothing, and will minimize the time his face is covered.

Carrying Your Baby

If you're like many new parents, yours may be the first newborn baby you've held. It can be intimidating — they seem so small and fragile. But like everything else, it will very quickly become second nature.

Support

The most important thing to remember when handling a baby is that you need to support his head and neck during the first few months of life until he gains better head control. When lifting a baby lying on his back, place one hand under his head and neck and the other under his

HOW TO: Care for Your Baby's Nails

A newborn baby's hands and feet are so small and cute that you might not even consider that the tiny nails require care. Some babies are even born with long nails, and although their nails are initially very soft, babies will very quickly scratch their own face, not to mention scratching you. Babies' nails grow quickly, so even if your baby's don't start out long, they will soon require a trim.

Invest in an inexpensive nail clipper or scissors made especially for babies, or a small nail file. These clippers or scissors have rounded tips designed to lessen the chance of injury.

Most parents find the process nerve-wracking at first, given a baby's tiny fingers, delicate skin, and squirmy disposition! You'll find, though, that if your baby is relaxed, his nails are so soft and small that the process is actually very quick and easy.

1. If you need a quick solution to your baby's scratching before you are prepared to cut his nails, place mittens or socks over his hands.
2. The best time to trim your baby's nails is when he's relaxed or even asleep. This time may often follow a feed, when he is lying content across your lap.
3. Make sure you have a good light source and two free hands. It's a job you can do either by yourself or with your partner's help.
4. With one hand, pull the fleshy tip of the finger back, away from the nail, to avoid snipping the skin.
5. With the other hand, simply clip the nail straight across.
6. If you do accidentally clip the skin, your baby may cry out, and there may even be a small amount of blood. Simply apply pressure to the cut with a clean tissue for a few minutes, and give your baby a cuddle. It's rarely serious. Rest assured that, at some point, it happens to every parent.
7. Don't forget about the toes! They're trimmed the same way, though you'll find that they don't grow as quickly as fingernails and thus need to be cut less often.
8. Trim your baby's nails routinely, every week or two. The frequency with which you'll need to care for your baby's nails is variable, as some nails grow faster than others.

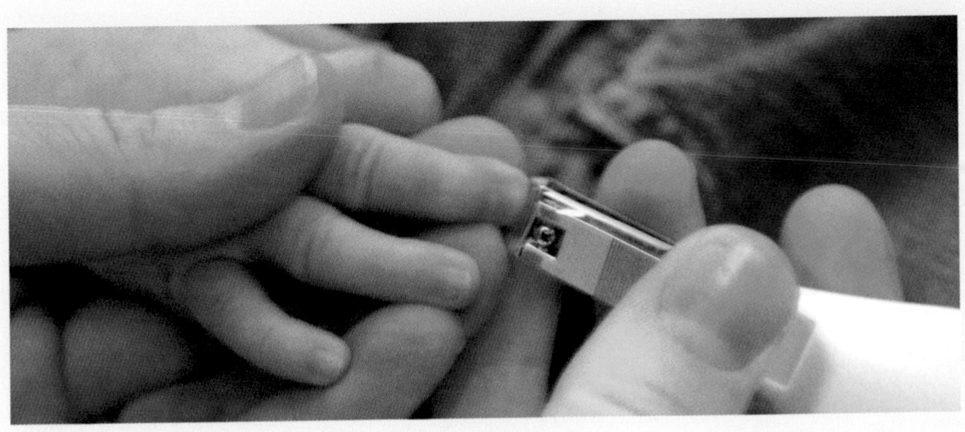

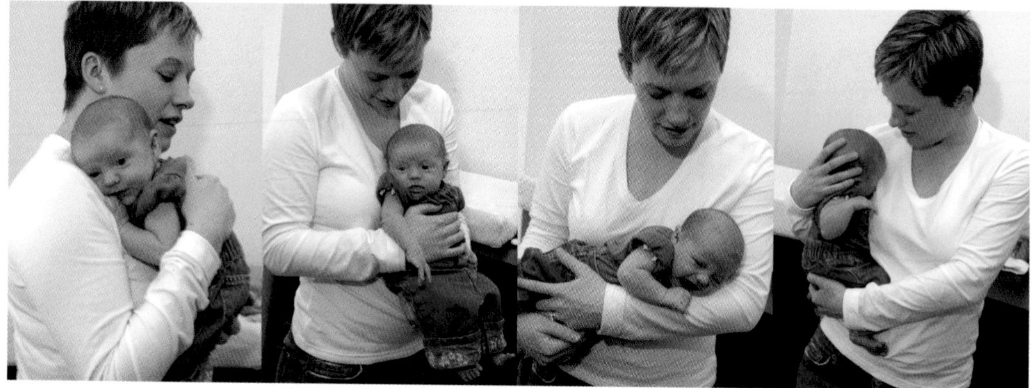

LEFT TO RIGHT: Shoulder hold; front-facing hold; tummy hold; hip hold.

bottom. Babies feel comforted when they're close to your body, so lean down, bringing yourself close to your baby as you lift him up to you. By the same token, lean down with him as you set him down, keeping your hands in place until he is settled, and then gently slip them out from under him.

DID YOU KNOW?

BABY CARRIERS

Many parents find that baby carriers or slings designed to hold a baby vertically against your front are invaluable for the first few months. Babies are snug up against you, and often fall asleep in this position. These carriers allow your arms to swing freely by your sides on a walk, to push a stroller with an older child, or to do things around the house.

Holds

There are several ways to carry your baby. As long as you have control over his head and neck, and you are both comfortable, go with whatever hold you both prefer! Babies can be carried over your shoulder, with one hand supporting his bottom and the other supporting his head. Some babies enjoy looking out at the world, achieved safely with a front-facing hold. Other babies, especially gassy ones, are comforted by resting on their tummies. As your baby gets older and has better head control, you may find that he is comfortable with his bottom resting against your hip and one of his arms tucked in around your back.

Frequently Asked Questions

My daughter is tongue-tied. Will this interfere with her ability to feed? Will I need to do anything about it?

"Tongue-tied" refers to a situation in which the tongue seems excessively tethered to the floor of the mouth by a thin strand of pinkish tissue, called the frenulum. It doesn't usually cause any problems unless it is so marked that the baby cannot protrude her tongue beyond her lower lip. In the rare case that treatment is truly needed, a simple release of the tongue can be achieved by snipping the frenulum. If your daughter is nursing well, it's best to leave things alone.

My baby has blue eyes. Will they remain that color?

Brown eyes invariably remain brown, but blue eyes may gradually change color over the first 8 or 9 months. Usually, deeply blue irises will remain blue permanently, while greenish blue irises are more likely to darken over time.

I have noticed a pinkish orange stain in many of my newborn's diapers. Should I be concerned? Is it blood?

This pinkish stain is quite common during the first week of life. It is not caused by blood; rather, it results when crystals in the urine are deposited onto the diaper. Although it is usually completely normal, it is often present in the concentrated urine that accompanies dehydration. Ask your health-care provider to weigh your baby; this is the best way to evaluate his state of hydration.

My newborn boy seems to have little breasts. Is that a sign of a hormonal or genetic problem?

Breast tissue is noticeable underneath the nipples in many boys and girls during the newborn period. This phenomenon is normal, caused by maternal hormones that were circulating around the time of your delivery. Don't worry: the "breasts" will eventually go away on their own.

My baby has a small bony lump in the middle of his chest. What should I do?

The lump is likely the slightly upturned triangular tip of the breast bone, called the xiphisternum. There isn't much fat or subcutaneous tissue at this site, so it often appears to be pushing up against the skin. Show the lump to your health-care provider at your next visit. If it's the xiphisternum, nothing further needs to be done.

My 1-week-old daughter sometimes seems to breathe very quickly, and then she actually stops for a few seconds. Does she have a breathing problem?

Not necessarily — or even likely. The normal breathing patterns of a newborn can seem quite irregular at times. What you are describing sounds like "periodic breathing," which is entirely normal. The breathing speeds up, then slows down, and sometimes even stops for a few seconds. Your daughter will outgrow this.

If, however, your daughter has to work very hard to breathe — sucking in the skin below or between her ribs, flaring her nostrils, or grunting with each breath — or if she stops breathing for more than 10 seconds or seems to be going a little blue around the mouth, you should definitely be concerned. True respiratory difficulty warrants immediate medical assessment.

My baby boy is uncircumcised. Should I be retracting the foreskin to clean around his penis?

Most people are unaware that the foreskin doesn't usually retract fully until a few years after birth. Many boys even have incomplete retraction of the foreskin into early adolescence. Washing the genital area with soap and water should be more than adequate cleansing. It is unwise to forcibly pull back on a foreskin that still naturally adheres to the underlying head of the penis.

CHAPTER 3

Feeding Your Baby

We highly recommend exclusive breast-feeding until 6 months of age, as do all health agencies. There is no doubt "breast is best." Nevertheless, both breast-feeding and formula-feeding are safe and nutritious ways to feed your baby. Do try to make your informed decision before your baby arrives. If you start by formula-feeding, it will be very difficult to change to breast-feeding if you wait too long, although you can switch from the breast to the bottle at any time.

Breast-Feeding or Formula-Feeding?

KEY POINT

You should not be made to feel guilty if breast-feeding is not possible for you. The decision is a personal one.

Today, breast-feeding is the most popular method of feeding, largely because medical research has shown that it has a number of advantages for both baby and mother. As a result, many mothers who choose to formula-feed feel anxiety and guilt about how other people will react — and perhaps criticize them. While breast milk is undoubtedly the best milk for newborn babies, infant formula is the next best thing. Formula is nutritionally sound, even though it does not offer the protective antibodies contained in breast milk. Infants will grow and develop appropriately and will be generally healthy when fed formula.

Recommended Feeding Options

The World Health Organization, the American Academy of Pediatrics and the Canadian Paediatric Society all recommend that babies be fed breast milk exclusively, with no other foods, until the age of 6 months. At that point, solid foods can be introduced. While the introduction of solid foods at 6 months is ideal, some parents do start solids at 4 months.

Continue to feed your baby breast milk or formula until she is about 1 year of age, at which time, if you are feeding her formula, you can switch to homogenized milk (3.25% whole cow's milk), which contains sufficient fat for the baby's growth. Of course, if your baby is known to have a specific allergy to cow's milk, non-dairy products will be needed: consult your doctor on which to try.

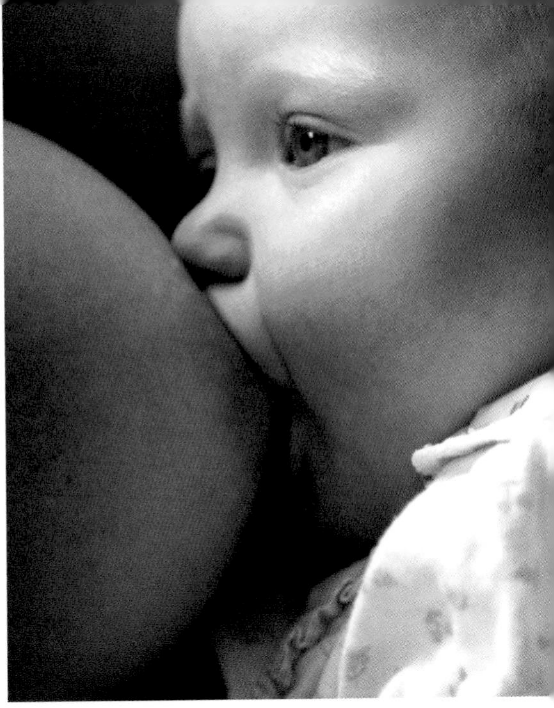

Cow's milk or any other kind of milk, such as goat's or almond milk, is not an appropriate choice for babies less than 1 year of age. Cow's milk has a significantly higher protein concentration than breast milk or infant formula. This puts undue stress on your baby's kidneys. The iron content in cow's milk is also low, which can place your baby at risk for iron-deficiency anemia.

Advantages of Breast-Feeding

New scientific evidence continues to emerge on a regular basis supporting the benefits of breast-feeding for your baby and for you.

For the Baby

- **Immune system improvement:** Breast-feeding will have a positive effect on your baby's immune system. Newborn babies' immune systems are immature, lacking the ability to fight off infections. Only at around 4 months does your baby's immune system really begin to mature. Breast milk provides your baby with your antibodies, to help fight infections. As a result, breast-fed babies have lower rates of gastrointestinal illness (such as diarrhea), ear infections, and respiratory infections.
- **Disease prevention:** Breast-feeding may decrease a child's risk of allergic disorders, notably asthma, as well as the risk of obesity, diabetes, cancer, high cholesterol levels, and sudden infant death syndrome (SIDS). More research in these areas is needed to determine the full extent of the benefits. From a growth and development standpoint, there is some evidence that breast-fed babies perform slightly better on cognitive development tests.

KEY POINT

Breast is best. There are advantages for both you and your baby, it is free, and it doesn't require any special preparation.

For the Mother

- **Uterine contractions:** Immediately following your baby's birth, breast-feeding will stimulate your uterus to contract. These contractions, much milder than the painful contractions of labor, decrease the risk of postpartum bleeding and help the uterus return to its original size. Your risk of breast and ovarian cancer has also been shown to decrease with breast-feeding.

KEY POINT

With the proper support and guidance, breast-feeding is a very enjoyable experience and a wonderful time to bond with your young baby.

- **Weight loss:** Breast-feeding burns approximately 500 calories a day. Studies show that mothers who breast-feed have an earlier rate of return to their pre-pregnancy weight.
- **Lactational amenorrhea:** Breast-feeding leads to lactational amenorrhea, increasing the time it will take for you to menstruate post-pregnancy and decreasing your chances of getting pregnant again soon after giving birth. But be aware that breast-feeding is by no means a reliable method of birth control!
- **Low cost:** Breast-feeding is free.

Disadvantages of Breast-Feeding

Although the advantages far outweigh the disadvantages, breast-feeding does have some minor drawbacks.

- **Insufficient breast milk supply:** In most cases, a mother is able to produce as much breast milk as her child needs. Occasionally, a mother may have an insufficient supply of breast milk and may need to supplement her breast-feeding with formula.
- **Isolation:** Breast-feeding requires a mother to be with her baby most of the time, which can be limiting at times. One way you can overcome this issue is by expressing breast milk, which can be fed to your baby in a bottle, allowing other caregivers an opportunity to feed the baby. This can be initiated after breast-feeding has been established.
- **Public attention:** Some women may be uncomfortable with the idea of breast-feeding in public, but many women become comfortable with it, finding ways to breast-feed discreetly. Privacy drapes can be purchased that help you cover up when feeding, or you can simply cover yourself with a receiving blanket. Some baby-friendly stores and restaurants even have a private room where you can feed your baby.
- **Complications:** Breast-feeding mothers may experience certain complications, such as sore nipples or yeast infections. These are generally easily treated.
- **Reduced sex drive:** Breast-feeding causes changes to vaginal secretions and to breast tissue, which may affect a woman's sex drive. These changes are not permanent, lasting only as long as you breast-feed.

DID YOU KNOW?

ANXIETY

In the first week or two, a nursing mother may experience significant anxiety about her ability to feed her baby. An encouraging partner and a skillful lactation consultant can provide invaluable reassurance that she, like most women, will succeed at nursing.

Advantages of Formula-Feeding

Despite the clear benefit of breast-feeding for infants, formula-feeding may have several possible attractions for families.

- **Partnership:** Formula-feeding may promote involvement of fathers, grandparents, other family members, and close friends who can help feed your baby formula from a bottle.
- **Flexibility:** Formula-feeding offers a little more flexibility for the mother because she does not need to be present for every feeding. Some mothers may need that space, either just to have a break or to do other activities, such as returning to work. This can also be achieved by pumping breast milk after breast-feeding is well established and bottle-feeding expressed breast milk.
- **Privacy:** Mothers do not usually feel uncomfortable when formula-feeding in social situations, nor do they feel limited in their outings with their baby.
- **Regularity:** Because formula takes a little longer to digest, formula-fed babies may not need to be fed as frequently as babies who are breast-fed.

Disadvantages of Formula-Feeding

- **Decreased immunity:** The biggest disadvantage of formula-feeding is that your baby will not receive the protective antibodies found in breast milk, which may help a baby fight infections.
- **Less convenience:** Because it requires advance planning and preparation, formula-feeding may not be as convenient as breast-feeding. Both at home and when going out, you need to ensure that you have formula, water for mixing it, and clean bottles and nipples on hand.
- **Slower return to pre-pregnancy state:** Many mothers dread the thought of how much activity it will take to get back to their pre-pregnancy state, especially after months of "eating for two." Formula-feeding does not burn the extra calories provided by breast-feeding.
- **Higher cost:** Formula-feeding can be expensive. While some formula preparations are less expensive than others, it will cost $1,500 to $2,000 a year ($125 to $165 a month) to feed your baby a regular formula. If your baby requires a specialized formula for digestive or allergic problems, it will cost considerably more.

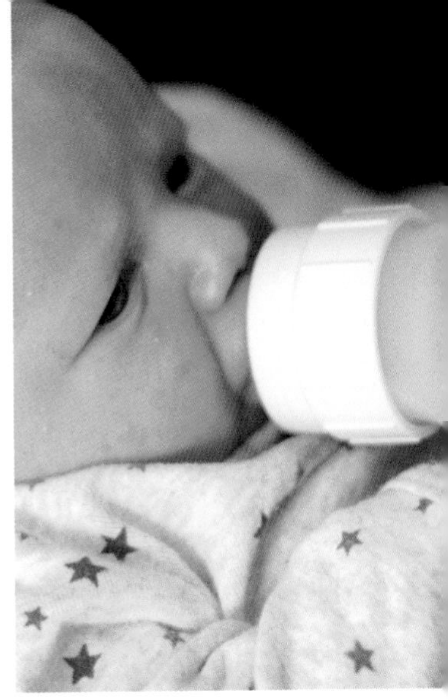

KEY POINT

With formula-feeding, you are able to tell exactly how much formula your baby is receiving. While this may be interesting information, remember that the best way to ensure that your baby is receiving appropriate nourishment is to monitor her growth in consultation with your health-care provider.

Getting Started with Breast-Feeding

So you have decided to breast-feed. Congratulations! It is a wise decision. To be successful at breast-feeding, there are a few things you will need to know. If you have spoken with any first-time mothers, they may have told you that breast-feeding is anything but natural at first. Both you and your baby will need to practice to get good at it. To make the process as effortless as possible, you need the proper support, knowledge, and equipment. With these three things in place, breast-feeding should be a lot easier.

Breast Milk Basics

Breast milk is based on "demand and supply" — the more your baby drinks, the more your breasts produce. Most women are able to produce more than enough breast milk to feed their baby, even if they have twins.

Your breasts are able to produce milk by the middle to end of your second trimester of pregnancy. You may notice your "first" milk, called colostrum, coming out of your nipples even before your child is born. Once you deliver your baby, your body releases a hormone called prolactin, which signals the glands in your breasts to start milk production. These milk glands both produce and store your breast milk.

The letdown reflex is triggered when your baby suckles at your breast, stimulating nerve endings that send a signal to your brain, which releases a hormone called oxytocin. (Pain, stress, and anxiety may decrease oxytocin levels.) Oxytocin signals your milk glands to release milk into your milk ducts, which lead out through the nipple and into your baby's mouth. Many women feel a tingling sensation in the nipple as this happens; others do not feel the reflex at all. In some women, the letdown reflex can be stimulated by other signals, such as hearing a baby cry or even looking at a picture of a baby.

Breast-Feeding Equipment

You may choose to breast-feed sitting in a comfortable chair or lying on a favorite couch or your bed. Wherever you end up, you should be completely relaxed so that your breast-feeding experience is as comfortable and enjoyable as possible.

DID YOU KNOW?

BREAST-FEEDING CLASSES AND CLINICS

If all goes well at the delivery, your baby will be breast-fed shortly after birth. Your nurse should be able to help you with breast-feeding. Ideally, you'll also be able to attend a class on breast-feeding while still in the hospital, before discharge. Your midwife, obstetrician, local hospital, public health unit, or La Leche League can provide information on beginners' classes or breast-feeding clinics being held in your neighborhood.

DID YOU KNOW?

LACTATION CONSULTANTS

Specialized support from a professional lactation consultant can be an invaluable resource when you start breast-feeding. Look for an International Board Certified Lactation Consultant (IBCLC) or a Registered Lactation Consultant (RLC).

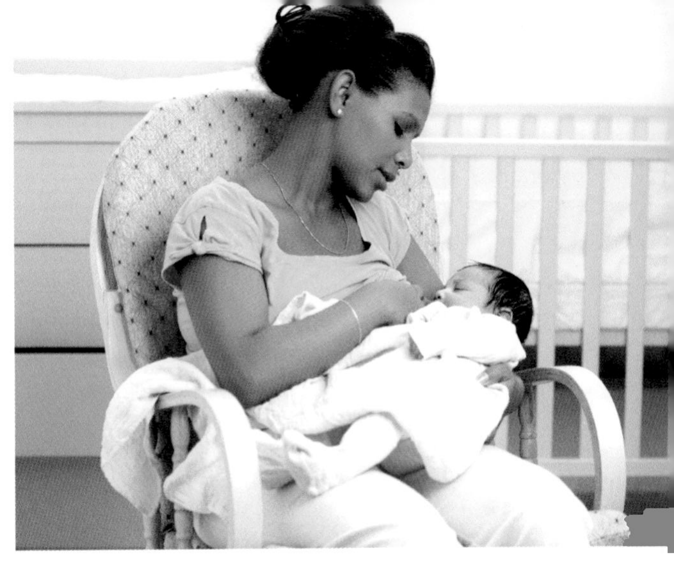

Pillow

If you are sitting up to feed, you will likely need a pillow. A special breast-feeding pillow, which can range in price from $30 to $100, may be preferred. Before you purchase one, try supporting your baby with a king-size pillow — you may find it works just as well.

Nursing Stool

When feeding in a chair, you may find you need to slouch for your baby to reach your breast, which can make feeding less comfortable. The solution is a nursing stool. Most women, unless they are tall or are sitting in a short chair, require a footrest. You can purchase a specialized nursing stool or simply place a large book under your feet to raise your knees, helping to lift the baby to your breast and prevent slouching.

Nursing Bras

Consider buying nursing bras so you don't have to undress when you are feeding. There are many styles, including bras with and without underwire. To prevent undue pressure on the breasts and secondary complications, make sure bras fit properly and are not too tight. Avoid purchasing too many before delivery, as your breast size is likely to change with engorgement and breast-feeding.

Breast-Feeding Positions

There are several different positions you can use to hold your baby while she is feeding. Personal preference varies, but the goal is constant: both you and your baby should be comfortable.

Most new mothers prefer to use the cross-cradle hold, and some may continue to use this position for the entire time they breast-feed. Others will transition to a cradle hold once they and their baby get the hang of breast-feeding. The best way to get comfortable with these positions is to practice and to have an experienced person help you. Make sure you have the proper equipment, such as pillows and a footrest, so that you are not slouching or straining.

KEY POINT

Whatever breast-feeding position you choose, your baby should always be brought to your breast. Avoid leaning in toward your baby.

Works Best For...

- Women learning to breast-feed
- Babies who have difficulty latching
- Little babies

Cross-Cradle Hold

1. Sit in a chair with your feet supported by a stool so that your legs are perpendicular to the floor, or sit cross-legged on the floor.
2. Hold the baby's back and head with the opposite arm and hand of the breast you intend to feed with. The arm holding the baby should be well supported by a large pillow.
3. The baby should be lying across you, with your tummies facing each other, and aligned so that the baby's nose is at your nipple.
4. Hold your breast with the hand on the same side.
5. Bring the baby to your breast using the latching technique described on page 61.

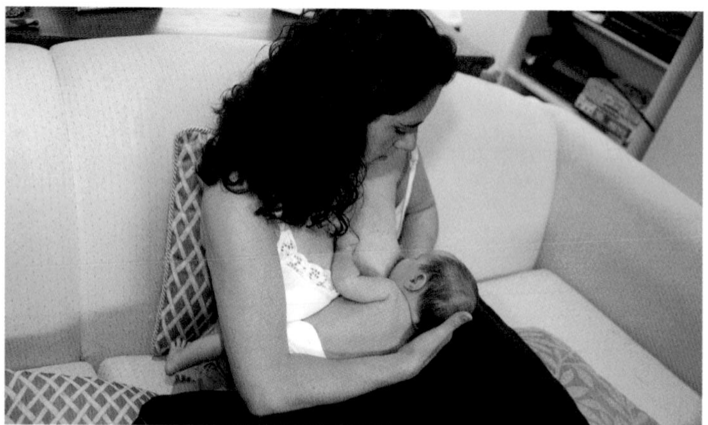

Cross-cradle hold

Works Best For...

- Women who are experienced at breast-feeding
- Babies who have no difficulty latching
- Feedings away from home, when you are without a pillow

Cradle Hold

1. Sit in a chair with your feet supported by a stool so that your legs are perpendicular to the floor, or sit cross-legged on the floor.
2. Hold the baby's back and head with your arm on the same side as the breast you intend to feed on. Your baby's head will lie cradled in your elbow. The arm holding the baby can be supported by a large pillow, but this is not necessary.
3. The baby should be lying across you, with your tummies facing each other and with the baby's nose at your nipple.
4. Hold your breast with the opposite hand.
5. Bring the baby to your breast using the latching technique described on page 61.

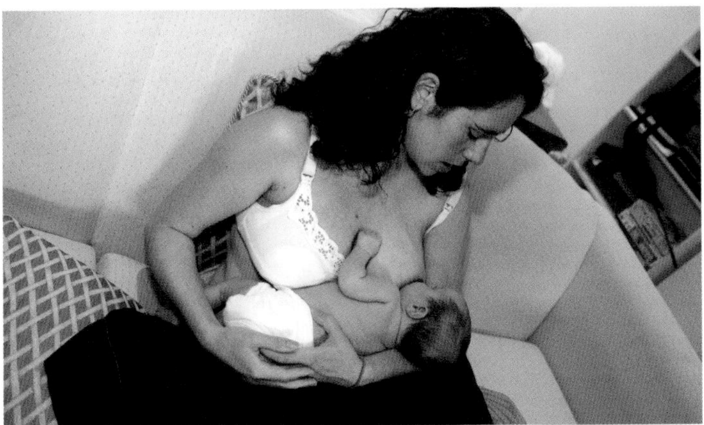

Cradle hold

Football Hold/Clutch Hold

1. Sit in a chair with your feet supported by a stool so that your legs are perpendicular to the floor, or sit cross-legged on the floor.
2. Hold the baby's back and head with your arm and hand on the same side as the breast you intend to feed on. The arm holding the baby should be well supported by a large pillow or two.
3. The baby's head should rest in your hand, and she should be lying somewhat flat on her back.
4. Hold your breast with the opposite hand.
5. Bring the baby to your breast using the latching technique described on page 61.

Works Best For...

- Feeding twins
- Little babies
- Women who have had Caesarean births
- Women with large breasts
- Women with flat or sore nipples

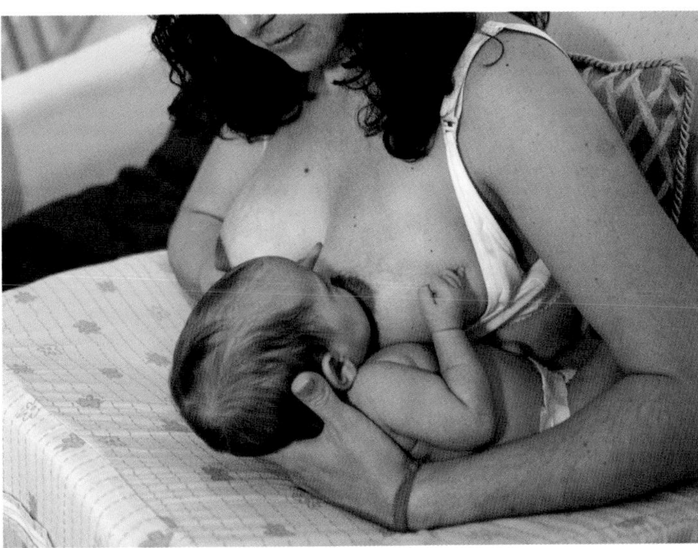

Football hold/clutch hold

Works Best For...

- Women who are uncomfortable sitting
- Women who have had Caesarean births
- Women with large breasts
- Women who want to rest while breast-feeding

Side-Lying Hold

1. Lie on your side with your baby lying on her side, facing you.
2. Draw your baby in toward your bottom breast using the arm on the same side.
3. With the opposite arm, position your bottom breast so that your baby can latch on.
4. Bring the baby to your breast using the latching technique described on page 61.
5. Once your baby is latched, you may move your bottom arm.

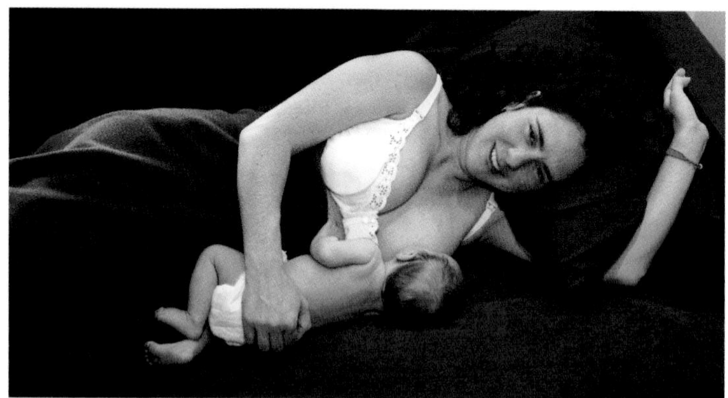

Side-lying hold

Feeding in the First 72 Hours

In the first few hours after delivery, your baby is very alert and ready to feed. Initiating breast-feeding at this time will pave the road for success in the future. The American Academy of Pediatrics recommends that the first feeding occur before the newborn is weighed and measured, treated with eye ointment, or given vitamin K.

KEY POINT

In the first few days, you may be concerned that your baby is not getting enough milk because your breast may not feel different before and after a feeding. Be assured that she is likely getting the appropriate, albeit rather small, amount of food she requires.

Colostrum

When you were pregnant, you may have noticed a sticky yellow substance leaking from your breasts. That substance is called colostrum. Colostrum is the "first" milk the breast produces until your mature "second" milk appears a few days later. Colostrum is very rich in nutrients and contains factors that boost your baby's immunity to infections. Because colostrum is so nutrient-dense, your baby needs only a very small amount at each feeding. In fact, during her first day of life, she needs only about 1 tablespoon (15 mL) of colostrum at each feeding; during her second day, her needs will be about double.

GUIDE TO: Latching Correctly

The latch is one of the most important elements of breast-feeding. An incorrect latch can result in significant breast-feeding problems. It's a good idea to ask for assistance from a trained lactation consultant or someone who has experience with breast-feeding.

There are eight main steps to a correct latch:

1. Hold your breast between your thumb and forefingers. Ensure that your hand is well behind the areola (the flat, colored part of the nipple) so that your hand does not get in the way of the baby's mouth. Gently compress your breast so that it is flattened out and similar to the shape of your baby's mouth.

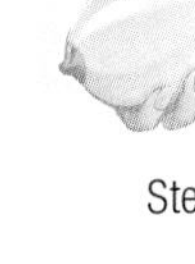

Step 1

2. Hold your baby so that her nose is at your nipple and her neck is very slightly tipped back.

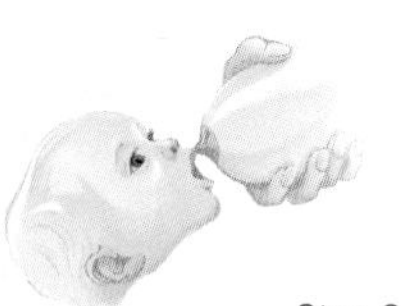

Step 3

3. Touch your baby's lip with your nipple to stimulate her to open her mouth.
4. Once your baby's mouth is open, pull her to the breast.

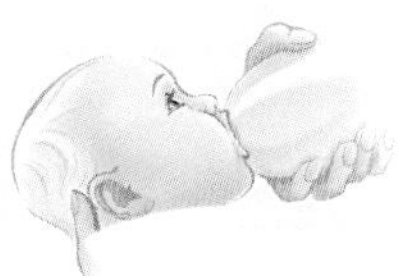

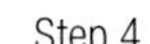

Step 4

5. Check the latch. If your baby is positioned correctly on your breast, much of your areola should be inside her mouth. Proportionately, more of the bottom of the areola will be in her mouth, and it will look like her chin is up against your breast. Both of your baby's lips should be flanged out – more simply, the baby should have "fish lips."

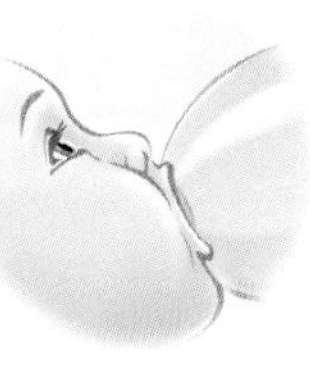

Step 5

6. If your baby falls asleep after a few minutes, gently squeeze your breast to help your milk flow. This will help your baby to start sucking again.

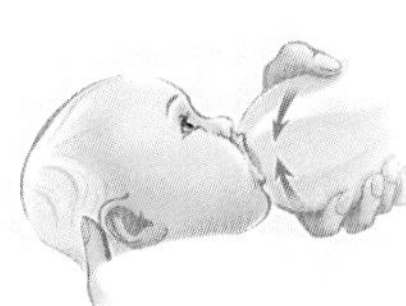

Step 6

7. If you feel pain or the positioning does not look correct, pull out the baby's upper or lower lip. If this doesn't rectify the problem, break the latch and try again.
8. To break the latch, slip your finger into the corner of your baby's mouth, between her gums, and break the seal her mouth has formed on your breast. Don't pull the baby off your breast without breaking the latch – this may cause you significant pain.

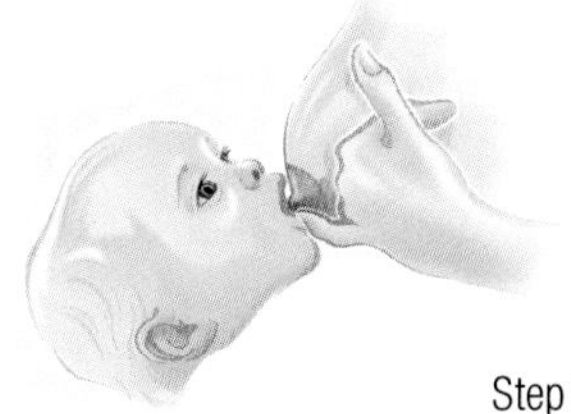

Step 8

DID YOU KNOW?

BREAST ENGORGEMENT

Most new mothers are able to breast-feed and will produce milk whether or not they intend to breast-feed. As a result, even women who choose not to breast-feed will have some initial engorgement, but this will subside. For women who choose to breast-feed, initial engorgement will subside if the baby is fed frequently from birth.

Frequent Feedings

After your baby's first feeding, she may become very tired and sleep for many hours. Even in these initial 24 to 48 hours, frequent feedings are essential once your baby has had a good rest. These early feedings will not only help your baby to excrete meconium, they will also stimulate your mature milk to come in and prevent engorgement.

Adequate Intake

Many new parents express concern that their newborn is not receiving an adequate intake of breast milk in the first few days of life. Most of the time, the colostrum is adequate. After all, a newborn's stomach is not much bigger than a cherry! Using the table on page 41, you can assess whether your baby's urine and stool output is sufficient.

▷ Newborn Hydration Red Flags

There are a few red flags to be aware of to ensure that your baby is adequately hydrated. If you note any of these, you and your baby should be seen by a health-care provider and a lactation consultant.

- Your baby is not voiding or is voiding insufficiently (see table on page 41).
- Your baby is not stooling or is stooling insufficiently.
- Your nipples are sore.
- Your baby is too sleepy to feed.
- Your baby has lost more than 7% of her birth weight by day 3.
- Your baby has lost more than 10% of her weight at any time.

Feeding Once Your Milk Comes In

You should produce mature milk within 2 to 5 days after the delivery of your baby. The second milk will be light in color and not sticky. Your breasts will also feel full, and, after your baby has fed, they will seem emptier. When your baby suckles at the breast, you will hear an audible swallowing noise.

Foremilk and Hindmilk

During the course of a single feed, the fat and caloric content of your breast milk changes. When your baby first suckles, she gets the foremilk: watery milk that is lower in fat and calories. Once she has fed for a few minutes, she will start to get the hindmilk, which has more fat and more calories.

The longer a baby feeds on one breast, the greater the chance that she will get hindmilk. Although hindmilk is richer in calories, which aid in growth and development, all of your milk is good for your baby.

Scheduled vs. Demand Feedings

Most babies need to be fed 8 to 12 times in a 24-hour period, but some may need to be fed less frequently, and others more. There are two main approaches mothers can use to figure out when to breast-feed: scheduled feedings and demand feedings.

With scheduled feedings, you feed your baby on a time-based schedule. For example, after consulting with your health-care provider, you might choose to feed her every 3 hours from the start of one feed to the start of the next.

With demand feedings, you feed the baby whenever she indicates that she is hungry. Learn to read your baby's hunger cues so that you can feed her before she starts crying — it can be very difficult to feed a screaming baby.

Waking Your Baby to Feed

In some situations, babies may be very sleepy and difficult to wake and feed. While you might be ecstatic that your newborn is sleeping for 6 hours in a row at night, you should be waking her up to feed if 4 hours have elapsed since the beginning of her last feeding.

To stimulate a sleepy baby to feed, try changing her diaper, taking off her sleeper, rubbing her back — anything that makes her a little uncomfortable and rouses her. If your baby is falling asleep on the breast, rub her under the chin to stimulate a suckle or rhythmically compress your breast with your hand to increase milk flow.

Later, once breast-feeding has been firmly established and your baby is gaining weight appropriately, waking her to feed is not necessary.

DID YOU KNOW?

BE FLEXIBLE

Regardless of the approach you adopt, be flexible. If you are feeding your child every hour because she demands it, it will be difficult for you to go anywhere or do anything. On the other hand, if your baby is on a schedule where she feeds every 3 hours, but is going through a growth spurt and is crying and rooting 2 hours after a feed, it is not fair to make her wait another hour before feeding her.

GUIDE TO: Your Baby's Hunger Cues

Learn to recognize these signs that your baby is hungry:

- **Waking:** Your baby may wake up or rouse from a deep sleep, stretching and perhaps yawning.
- **Rooting:** Your baby may start rooting: nuzzling toward your chest or the chest of anyone holding her.
- **Fist sucking:** Your baby may suck on her fists or make sucking motions with her mouth.
- **Crying:** If you don't notice her other cues, your baby may start to cry. One word of caution: a crying baby is not necessarily a hungry baby. When offered the breast, most babies, hungry or not, will suckle, and they will stop crying because suckling is soothing. Learning to read your baby's hunger cues will help you know when your baby is hungry and when she is crying for another reason (see Interpreting Crying, page 99).

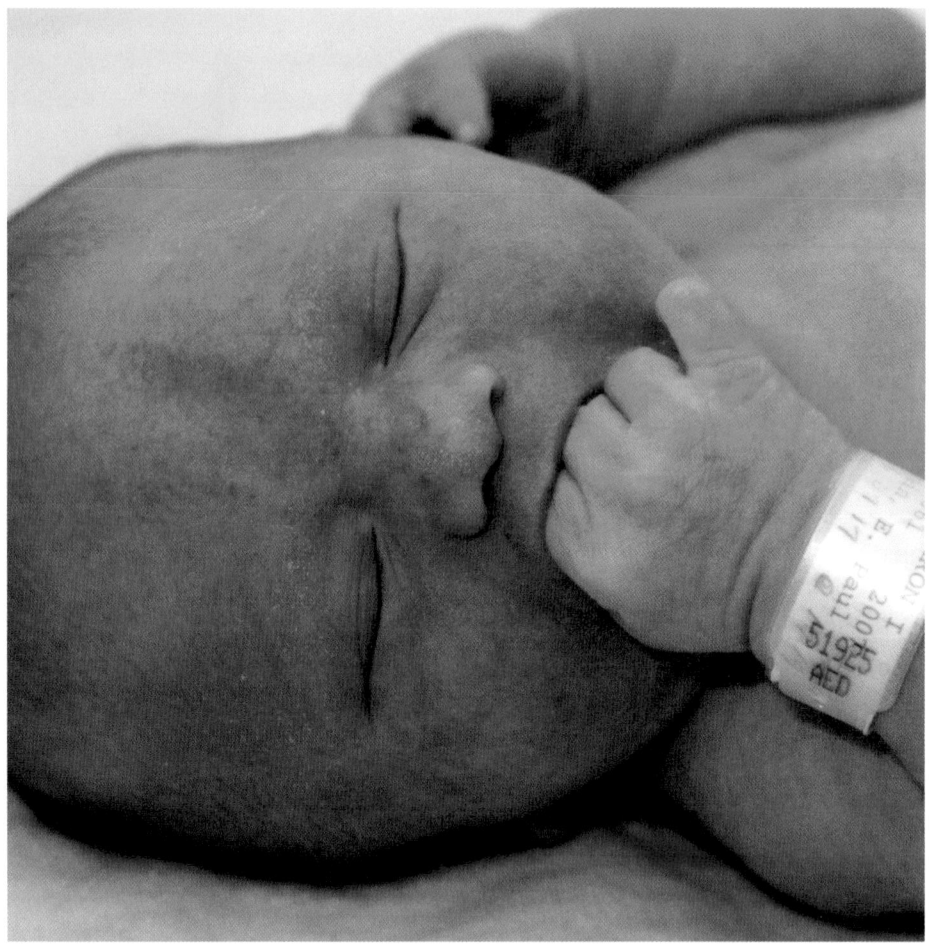

Feeding Duration

Like adults, babies can be fast or slow eaters. Milk supply also varies among mothers: some have a very fast flow of milk, while others have a slower flow, making feeding last longer. Some general guidelines will help you ensure that each feeding is adequate for your baby:

- Let your baby feed for as long as she wants to. You will know she is feeding because you will see her jaw moving and hear her swallow. Once she is finished, she may fall asleep on the breast or she may pull off the breast.
- During a feeding, feed your baby from both breasts. Once she is done feeding on one breast, break her latch and move her to the other. If she is sleepy, you may need to rouse her before she will latch on to your other breast. Alternatively, if she is still hungry, she may latch on eagerly.
- Start each feed on the opposite breast than you last started on. This will help keep your milk supply steady. It is common for babies to drink more from the first breast than from the second. In fact, some babies may not want to feed on the second breast.

Growth Spurts

As your baby grows, you will encounter many changes in her feeding requirements. At 3 weeks, 6 weeks, and 3 months of age, babies commonly go through a growth spurt. Growth spurts can last 4 to 5 days. At these times, it will seem like your baby wants to feed constantly. Your milk supply will increase with the more frequent feedings, so resist the temptation to supplement your breast milk with formula.

Cluster Feeding

Another common feeding variation is called cluster feeding, when your baby wants to feed more often than usual. This may occur during a growth spurt or on a more regular basis at a specific time of day — for example, in the evenings, before bedtime. Not all babies cluster feed, and unlike a growth spurt, it may not stop in 4 to 5 days.

Feeding Beyond the Newborn Months

Many mothers wonder how often they should breast-feed their baby after the newborn period (beyond 3 months

DID YOU KNOW?

WEIGHT LOSS

Following birth, it is common for a baby to lose some weight. A loss of 7% to 10% of your baby's original birth weight is considered acceptable. For example, if your baby weighs 7.7 pounds (3.5 kg) at birth, an initial loss of up to 0.5 pound (0.25 kg) is no cause for concern. When the loss is greater than 7% to 10%, an evaluation of the baby and the feeding method by a health-care provider is generally warranted to ensure that the baby is feeding appropriately.

of age). Many authorities recommend breast-feeding on demand at this stage, but new mothers often want to maintain a feeding schedule and sometimes feel that they can't pick up on all their baby's cues.

For babies who are gaining weight and thriving, it can be helpful to use the feeding schedule for formula-fed babies as a guide (see table, page 81). Breast milk is digested more rapidly than formula, so it makes sense to breast-feed babies at the upper limit of these recommendations, or slightly more frequently than bottle-fed babies. By following these guidelines and assessing your baby's cues for hunger, you should be able to create a feeding schedule that fulfills your baby's needs.

Common Breast-Feeding Problems

Initiating breast-feeding is a learning process both for you and your baby. With practice, breast-feeding soon becomes fairly straightforward. If you do encounter problems, knowing how to assess and manage them is important for your health and the welfare of your baby. Listed below are some common problems and their suggested treatments. Seek care from a health-care provider or specialist in breast-feeding if the problem persists.

Treating Common Breast-Feeding Problems

DIAGNOSIS	SIGNS AND SYMPTOMS	COMMON TREATMENT
Sore and/or cracked nipples	• Red, dry nipples • Visible cracks in nipples • Pain with breast-feeding, usually most severe when baby first starts to nurse • Nipple is "pinched" when the baby comes off the breast	• Ensure that your baby is latching correctly — an incorrect latch is the usual cause of sore or cracked nipples. • After feeding, express a few drops of breast milk onto your nipple and let it dry. • Make sure your nipples always have a chance to dry after feeding. • Wear breathable breast pads. • Use a breast shield between feeds if needed. • Apply lanolin ointment to nipples after each feed. • Do not apply creams or lotions that you need to remove prior to feeding. • When bathing, use only water (no soap) on breasts.

DIAGNOSIS	SIGNS AND SYMPTOMS	COMMON TREATMENT
Leaking nipples	• Breast milk leaks out of nipples and onto bra or clothing when baby is not feeding	• None — this is a natural occurrence for some women. • To prevent leakage onto your bra and clothing, use breathable breast pads to collect milk.
Engorgement Breasts become too full with milk. Commonly occurs when milk first comes in or if feedings are missed.	• Breasts are extremely full and hard • Breasts may hurt when touched • Breasts are very warm • Areolas are hard, difficult for baby to latch on	• Express breast milk frequently to relieve the pressure (preferably with a pump). • Breast-feed more frequently. • Apply warm compresses prior to feeding. • Apply cold compresses for severe engorgement between feeds. Massage your breasts, starting from your armpit and going down to your nipple, prior to feeding or expressing. • Consider pain medication as required (ibuprofen or acetaminophen).
Blocked duct One of the ducts that your milk flows through has become plugged.	• Usually localized to one breast • One section of the breast is red, hard, and often painful • A lump may be felt	• Feed frequently — your baby's sucking will help unblock the duct. • Start feeding on the side that is blocked. • Try feeding your baby in a different position and try to position her so that her jaw is on the side of the blocked duct. • Apply moist heat to the affected area. • Massage the affected area. • Monitor a blocked duct very closely — it can lead to mastitis if not treated.
Mastitis Bacterial infection of the breast tissue, usually localized to one breast.	• Pain or swelling in the breast, similar to a blocked duct • Redness of the breast tissue around the painful site • Fever and other flu-like symptoms	• Try treatments for a blocked duct, but if symptoms persist for more than 24 hours, seek immediate medical attention and treatment with antibiotics. • Continue to breast-feed regularly. This infection does not affect the quality of the breast milk, and feeding may help treat the mastitis — abrupt cessation of breast-feeding will exacerbate the problem. • To prevent mastitis, avoid pressure on the breast (from a poorly fitting bra, for example); feed your baby regularly; and ensure that she has a good latch and is draining the breast effectively.

DIAGNOSIS	SIGNS AND SYMPTOMS	COMMON TREATMENT
Yeast infection May follow antibiotic use in mother or baby.	• Deep, shooting pain or burning while breast-feeding that lasts for the entire feed, and even after the feed in some instances • Pain and very sensitive nipples while not breast-feeding • Breasts may or may not show any physical signs, such as swelling or discoloration • Baby may or may not have white patches (thrush) in her mouth or a persistent diaper rash	• Ensure that your baby is latching correctly — an incorrect latch will increase your pain. • Continue to breast-feed regularly. This infection does not affect the quality of the breast milk. • Keep breasts dry and, if possible, expose them to the air as much as possible. • Do not use breast pads with plastic lining or wear a bra that traps moisture around the nipple. • Change your bra daily. • If the baby has a pacifier, sterilize it daily. • See your health-care provider: topical treatments, such as clotrimazole, are generally used first. • Treat the baby with a topical antifungal (for example, nystatin). She may have oral thrush.

Expressing and Storing Breast Milk

Expressed breast milk allows a baby to feed from a bottle or cup while still receiving the best possible nutrition. Expressing milk offers many advantages for mothers, too. They get some free time, and it allows for continuation of breast-feeding after they return to work. Expressing milk may also provide a mother with engorged breasts some relief, or it can help to increase milk supply in certain situations. In addition, other family members have an opportunity to bond with the baby while feeding her your breast milk.

KEY POINT

Never squeeze the nipple — this will occlude the milk ducts, and milk will not be able to come out.

Expressing Breast Milk

There are two basic ways to express breast milk: manually (using your hands) and mechanically (using a pump). While pumps have become increasingly popular, this is an individual decision, and you may find that manual expression works for you.

Expressing Milk Manually

Manual milk expression can be done anywhere. It is a learned skill — your ability to express milk this way will improve with practice.

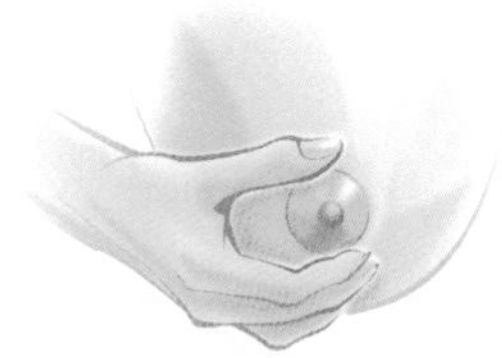

Step 3

1. Wash your hands.
2. Select a container to hold the milk. A container with a large opening and a pouring spout is best. A large measuring cup works perfectly. Wash it with warm soapy water, then rinse.
3. Hold your hand in a "C" shape and cup the breast closest to the hand. Make sure your thumb is opposite from your index finger and middle finger, about 1 inch (2.5 cm) away from the nipple.
4. Gently pull your thumb and fingers back in toward your chest.
5. Squeeze your thumb and fingers together and move them forward toward the areola.
6. Continue to do this until the milk supply slows down (it starts dripping rather than squirting). You may need to change your hand's position, moving it around your breast.

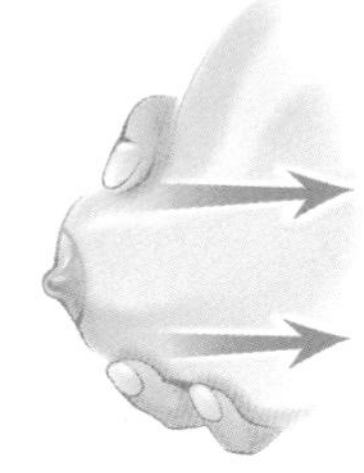

Step 4

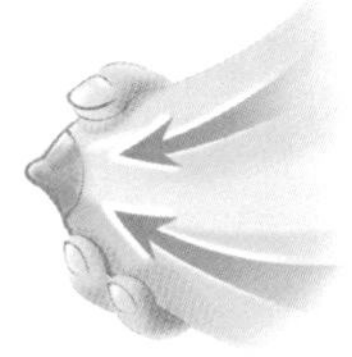

Step 5

Expressing Milk Mechanically

There are three kinds of pumps you can purchase to express breast milk: a hand pump, a small single-breast battery-operated pump, and a large electric (or battery-operated) dual breast pump. Each has its benefits and is suitable for a different situation. Wash the pump in hot soapy water after every use. Be sure to check the manufacturer's instructions on cleaning. If you plan on using it while out of the house, remember to pack some cleaning supplies.

Storing Expressed Breast Milk

Once you have pumped breast milk, you will need to store it correctly to prevent contamination and nutrient loss. Expressed milk should be refrigerated or frozen unless you plan on feeding it to the baby shortly after pumping.

There are many different opinions on how to store breast milk — the "best" way has yet to be scientifically

KEY POINT

An electric pump is the best way to obtain large volumes of breast milk quickly. It is the method of choice for situations that require exclusive feeding with expressed breast milk.

Breast Milk Pumps

TYPE OF PUMP	AVERAGE COST	USES, DISADVANTAGES AND BENEFITS
Hand pump	\$30 to \$70	• Good for occasional pumping (once a week or less) • Can pump only one breast at a time • Requires a small amount of hand strength to operate • Easy to travel with • Best results once milk is established (may not work as well immediately following birth)
Small single-breast battery-operated pump	\$80 to \$130	• Good for periodic pumping (once a week or less) • Can pump only one breast at a time • Battery-operated • Easy to travel with
Large electric (or battery-operated) dual breast pump	\$100 to \$500	• Good for frequent pumping (daily use) • Can pump both breasts simultaneously, taking less time to pump • Larger than single-breast pumps • More cumbersome to travel with • Best results if trying to establish volume

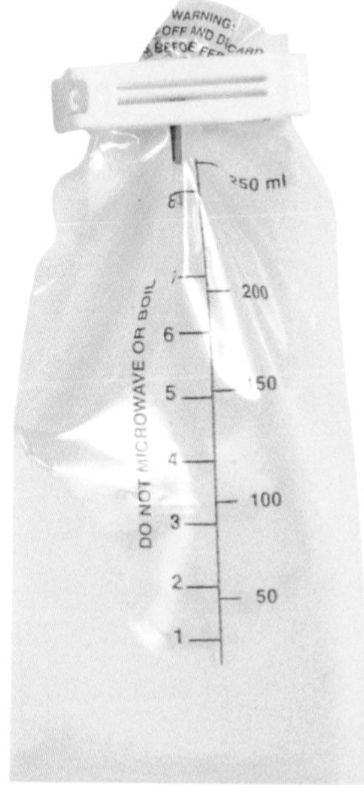

A breast milk storage bag.

determined. In the meantime, here are some guidelines that will help you store it safely:

- Purchase clean glass or plastic containers with tight lids.
- If you choose to store your milk in plastic bags, use breast milk storage bags designed for this purpose. Regular bottle liners or plastic bags may destroy some of your milk's protective antibodies.
- Always date the container so you can keep track of how long you have been storing the milk.
- Store milk in small amounts (2 to 4 oz/60 to 120 mL) so that you don't end up wasting it.
- Don't add unfrozen milk to previously frozen milk. This may promote the growth of bacteria.
- Never refreeze milk once it is thawed.
- Store expressed breast milk in the refrigerator for 3 to 8 days; in the freezer of a one-door refrigerator for up

to 2 weeks; in the freezer of a two-door refrigerator for up to 3 months; or in a deep freezer for 6 to 12 months. Refrigerated or frozen breast milk often separates, with the fatty component on top; this is perfectly normal, just stir fat back in.

Breast Pumping Difficulties

For some women, expressing breast milk is very simple, while others have more difficulty. The first few times, it may seem like you pump forever and get only a very small amount of milk, perhaps just ¼ to ½ ounce (7.5 to 15 mL). While this can be frustrating, it is completely normal. It doesn't mean you have less milk, nor is it representative of what your baby is getting during regular feeds.

KEY POINT

Don't worry if your expressed milk has a slight yellowish or even bluish tinge. This is normal.

Letdown

Some women find it difficult to achieve a letdown response using a pump. To make the process more productive, be sure you are in a warm, comfortable place when you are pumping. You may want to put warm compresses on your breasts or take a shower before pumping. Also, make sure you are in a quiet, private environment free of disruptions. Having your baby present, or a picture of your baby, may help you achieve letdown more easily.

Take care to choose the best time to pump, coordinated with your regular feeding schedule and your milk supply. Your milk supply fluctuates during the day and night. Most women find their breasts are fullest in the middle of the night and in the early morning, so you could try pumping when you first wake up to get the best volume.

Pumping Pain

Pumping should not be painful, but if you pump for long periods at a time, you may feel pain. Short, frequent pumping sessions may be more rewarding and less traumatic to your sensitive breast tissue. If you are using an electric pump, you may be tempted to increase the pressure of the pump to shorten the time it takes to pump or to pump more milk. Be wary when increasing the pressure: do it very slowly and stop if you feel pain — it may result in sore or cracked nipples. You may end up having more difficulty achieving letdown because you anticipate pain when using the pump.

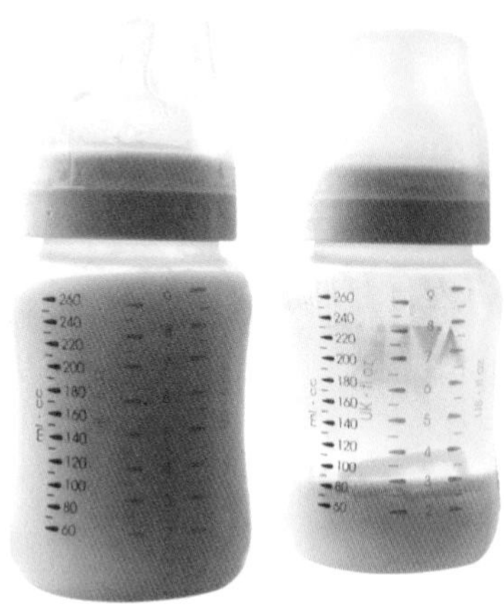

A yellowish or even bluish color is normal for expressed milk.

Introducing the Bottle

Once breast-feeding is well established, by the time your baby is 4 to 6 weeks of age, you may want to try expressing your milk and offering her a bottle. How frequently you choose to offer the bottle is up to you. However, infants prefer a routine, so if you don't routinely offer them a bottle, they may not want to take it when you want them to.

Offer your child a bottle of breast milk every few days while you are breast-feeding so she will start to accept the bottle as a substitute. You may have another family member feed her the bottle, depending on your situation. Some babies may not want to take a bottle from their mother because they prefer to breast-feed from her. Now is a good time to let Dad have a hand in feeding.

KEY POINT

Once your baby has finished feeding, discard any milk left in the bottle to prevent bacterial contamination.

Preparing the Milk and the Bottle

If you are feeding breast milk you have just pumped, no preparation of the milk is required. If you are feeding milk that was frozen, thaw it by placing it in the refrigerator or in a bowl of warm water. Do not thaw or warm up breast milk in a microwave. Too much heat can damage the proteins and vitamins in breast milk, and hot spots from uneven heating can scald a baby's mouth.

Clean the bottle before putting milk in it, and give the bottle a gentle shake after filling it: expressed milk separates so that the fat lies on top, and shaking will redistribute it.

Weaning Your Child

Most people believe weaning means the process of stopping breast-feeding, but it is more accurately described as the process of starting to feed your child something other than breast milk, such as infant formula or cereal. The current recommendation is to breast-feed exclusively until your baby is 6 months old and then start introducing solid foods along with the breast milk. Be sure to introduce iron-fortified foods; infant iron stores start to become depleted between 4 and 6 months of age.

If a baby is weaned off breast milk prior to 12 months of age, the milk feedings should be replaced with iron-fortified infant formula. At 12 months of age, 3.25% cow's milk may be introduced, and at 24 months, it can be changed to 2% cow's milk.

HOW TO: Wean Your Child

The best way to wean a child off the breast is slowly — it will be easier on both of you. However, there is no "correct" number of days to wait between dropped feedings. You might drop a feeding every few days, weeks, or months. Some women choose only partial weaning, continuing to breast-feed their baby at certain feeding times (for example, morning and night).

To begin weaning, follow these steps:

1. Determine your baby's least favorite feeding time.
2. For this dropped feeding, give her formula or milk (depending on her age) by bottle or cup.
3. If your child initially refuses the bottle, keep trying, or have another family member try to give this feeding.
4. Once this feeding is going well — after, say, a few days to a week — substitute another bottle or cup feed.
5. Continue dropping feedings until you have reached your goal — partial or full wean.

Weaning should not be abrupt unless there is an emergency situation — for example, if a mother needs to start treatment for a disease. If you need to wean your child quickly, you may suffer engorgement, blocked ducts, or mastitis.

Getting Started with Formula-Feeding

Feeding your baby formula takes additional preparation time, but it means other people can help you. You get a much-needed break while your partner or another caregiver has an opportunity for some bonding time with the baby.

The use of formula also requires extra financial outlay. While regular powdered formula can be costly, liquid concentrate or ready-to-feed formula can be even more so.

Formula itself is not the only expense: you'll also need some equipment.

KEY POINT

If you have difficulty getting your baby to take a bottle, never force her. Continue to offer her the bottle from time to time, or have another person offer it to her until she accepts this way of feeding.

Formula-Feeding Equipment

If you plan on formula-feeding your baby (or feeding her breast milk by bottle), you will need to buy bottles, nipples, and, in some cases, a sterilizer.

Bottles

There are many types of bottles available on the market — plastic bottles, glass bottles, bottles with disposable liners, straight bottles, angled bottles, venting bottles, and anti-colic bottles. While some research has been done on the merits of various bottles, there is not enough evidence to recommend one particular type over another. The choice is one of personal preference.

GUIDE TO: Choosing a Bottle

Consider these questions when choosing a bottle for your baby:

- Is it made of plastic or glass? If it is breakable, does this concern you?
- What do the instructions say about how to sterilize it?
- Is it microwave-safe for sterilization?
- Does it have a wide mouth (which makes it easier to clean)?
- Does it have a lot of little pieces to clean?
- Will you need to buy disposable liners?
- Will your baby be able to hang on to it when she gets older?

Nipples

Once you have chosen a bottle, you face another decision: what nipples should you buy for it? Manufacturers of certain nipples profess that their nipple is more like the human nipple or helps to reduce colic, but there is limited evidence for these claims. Choose a nipple that is easy to clean and that works with the bottle you prefer.

Nipples are commonly made of silicone or latex. Silicone nipples are typically (but not always) firmer than latex nipples; for this reason, new babies may prefer latex nipples. Silicone nipples are clear in color, which makes them easier to clean; latex nipples are usually brown.

Nipples also come in different shapes: standard nipples, long rounded-tip nipples, nubbin nipples, tricot nipples, flat-tipped orthodontic nipples, preemie nipples, and specialty nipples (such as Haberman nipples).

Nipples break down, get worn, and need replacing, so be sure to monitor the quality of the nipples you are using and replace them if they are dirty and cannot be cleaned, if the holes become too large, or if the material starts to break down.

DID YOU KNOW?

FLOW RATES

Different nipples have different flow rates. Every manufacturer has its own system for grading the flow. Some use numbers, while others grade their nipples as slow, medium, or fast. For newborn babies, choose nipples with a slow flow rate. As your baby grows, increase the flow rate (which means purchasing new nipples) according to manufacturer guidelines.

Sterilization Equipment

Water and equipment used to feed babies should be sterilized until the babies are 3 to 4 months old. This is the age when babies typically start to pick things up and put them in their mouth; it is also when their developing immune system allows them to fight off infections more effectively. Sterilization is no longer warranted by this age.

In fact, many experts feel that, in developed countries with safe drinking water, it is probably not necessary to boil the water used to reconstitute formula. And modern dishwashers do a fine job of cleaning bottles and nipples, especially if the nipples are scrubbed first.

Still, you may choose to sterilize formula water and bottles. The least expensive way to do this is to immerse the equipment in a pot of boiling water for at least 5 minutes. But there are faster, safer, and more efficient ways to sterilize equipment. Electric steam sterilizers plug into an outlet and turn off automatically when finished. Sterilizers that you put into the microwave for a few minutes are available, as are containers that hold bottles and nipples in position in the dishwasher.

Water Safety

Even if you sterilize the water you use to reconstitute formula, you need to consider its safety. Some water sources, such as well water, contain substances that may be harmful to small babies, such as nitrites, arsenic, and heavy metals. Before using well water to mix formula, have it tested to ensure that it is safe.

Many older houses contain lead pipes that can leave sediment in your water. Hot water is more likely to contain sediment. It is best to turn on your cold water tap and let it run for 2 minutes to clear any contaminants. Then you can collect the water you will use to mix formula. You should let the water run even if you plan on boiling it.

KEY POINT

Added fluoride in tap water is fine for your baby. In fact, if the water supply in your area does not contain fluoride, your health-care provider may recommend that you supplement with fluoride.

Choosing a Formula

It can be tough to determine the right formula to buy. When you're standing in the store, all the options you're faced with can be daunting. Relax. Buying formula is like buying a carton of milk: although every company that makes formula claims that their product is unique, they all basically taste the same.

Formula is offered in several different bases — cow's milk, soy, and protein hydrolysate, for example. Once you determine the type appropriate for your baby (formula based on cow's milk will usually do), you just need to choose from one of the many brands.

Formulas

BASE	CHARACTERISTICS	USE
Cow's milk	• Made with cow's milk, but it has been significantly changed so that the composition of fat and protein is similar to that of breast milk • Best taste • Average cost • Not all brands are iron-fortified; choose one that is	• Appropriate for almost all healthy full-term infants, except those with a true allergy to cow's milk protein or a strong family history of allergy to cow's milk protein
Soy	• Made from soybeans • Not currently recommended for routine use unless there is a reason why cow's milk protein formulas are not appropriate • Average taste • Average cost • All brands are iron-fortified	• Not generally suitable for children with an allergy to cow's milk protein, because it is estimated that 50% will be allergic to soy as well (use a casein hydrolysate formula instead) • Suitable for infants whose parents wish to maintain a strict vegetarian or vegan diet • Generally lactose-free, so can be given to infants with lactose intolerance • Some varieties may be suitable for infants whose parents wish to maintain a halal or kosher diet — check formula containers when purchasing to verify
Lactose-free cow's milk	• Based on cow's milk, but free of lactose • Does not taste as good as regular cow's milk formulas • More expensive than regular cow's milk formulas	• Suitable for infants who are lactose-intolerant (which is quite rare)

BASE	CHARACTERISTICS	USE
Protein hydrolysate Whey hydrolysate or casein hydrolysate, also called hypoallergenic	• Whey hydrolysates are broken into quite large proteins; casein hydrolysates are broken into very small proteins and can be used in infants with allergic disorders • Casein hydrolysates do not taste good, but are well accepted by younger infants, whose sense of taste is not yet well developed • Casein hydrolysate formulas are more expensive • More costly than regular cow's milk or soy-based formulas	• *Whey hydrolysate formulas:* Not suitable for children with an allergy to cow's milk protein; sometimes recommended for infants with gastroesophageal reflux disease • *Casein hydrolysate formulas:* Suitable for infants with a diagnosed allergy to cow's milk protein; casein hydrolysate formulas should be used only if recommended by a pediatric health-care provider • Used when an infant has one of various conditions that cause damage to the lining of the bowel, making it more difficult to digest and absorb regular formulas
Amino acid	• Made from amino acids • Poor taste • Extremely costly	• Used in special medical situations, such as with severe malabsorptive conditions • Used only when recommended by a pediatric health-care provider
Follow-up formulas	• Cow's milk or soy • Can be used from 6 to 12 months and beyond • Marketed as good for your baby because they contain higher levels of calcium and iron • Superior to cow's milk for a baby less than 1 year old, but have not been proven superior to starter formulas • Best taste • Less expensive than basic starter formulas	• Suitable for children 6 months and older, if the parent wishes

Iron Fortification

Make sure the formula you choose is iron-fortified. All soy-based formulas are fortified with iron, but not all cow's milk formulas are. Although regular formulas do have some iron, it is insufficient to meet the baby's needs. Contrary to popular belief, iron-fortified formulas have not been shown to cause constipation, but they will help prevent iron-deficiency anemia.

Formula Preparations

Cow's milk and soy-based formulas come in three standard preparations: powder, liquid concentrate, and ready-to-feed. All provide adequate nutrition for your baby.

Formula Preparations

PREPARATION	ADVANTAGES	DISADVANTAGES
Powder	• Least expensive • Tin of powder lasts for up to 1 month once opened • Tin does not need to be refrigerated	• Can be messy when out in public; need a special container to carry it • Need clean (or sterile) water to mix with • Risk of incorrect measurement of powder
Liquid concentrate	• Very easy to mix • Very easy to measure • Less expensive than ready-to-feed	• If going out, need to premix bottle • Need to mix more than one bottle at a time; otherwise, you end up discarding and wasting the rest of the concentrate, as it makes more than one bottle • Need clean (or sterile) water to mix with • Once opened, good for only 48 hours and must be refrigerated
Ready-to-feed	• Most convenient: just open, pour into bottle, and feed • No need to have clean (or sterile) water to mix with	• Most expensive

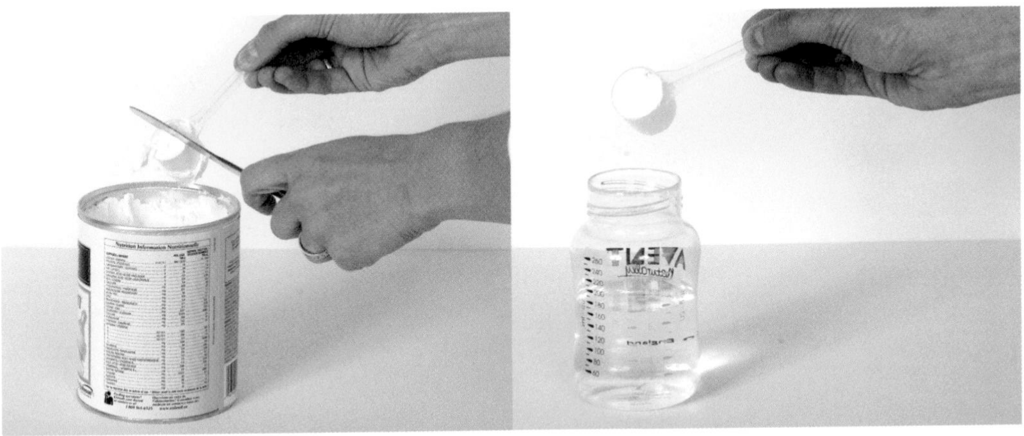

Follow the directions on the tin precisely.

Preparing the Bottle

The correct way to prepare your baby's bottle is to closely follow the directions provided by the formula company. While most directions are similar, there may be slight differences between brands, so it is important to read the instructions carefully.

Powder and liquid concentrate preparations should be mixed with water prior to feeding. Too little water can concentrate the formula, making it difficult for your baby's body to digest and putting undue stress on the kidneys. Too much water decreases the concentration of the formula, as well as the calories, putting your child at risk for inadequate growth and electrolyte disturbances.

KEY POINT

Unless you are directed by a health-care provider to mix the formula differently, you should follow the directions exactly as they appear on the can.

Warming Bottles

There is no need to warm a baby's bottle. Babies will drink what they are given and will get used to a warm or cold bottle. If you always warm your baby's bottle, she might not take one that is cold or at room temperature. This may prove difficult if you find yourself with a screaming hungry baby at a time when you are not able to warm the bottle.

If you do choose to warm the bottle, be cautious about how you do it, to avoid burning your baby's mouth. Heat the formula until it is lukewarm. To test the temperature, shake a few drops onto the inner part of your wrist. If it feels neither cold nor hot, then it is lukewarm and should not be heated further. Always mix the contents of the bottle before serving it to your baby to ensure an equal temperature throughout. Do not use a microwave to warm a bottle — microwave heat is very uneven. When a bottle of milk is heated in a microwave, it may feel cool to the touch on the outside; however, there may be very hot areas of liquid on the inside.

Storage

Once you have mixed the formula, you may or may not be able to store it. Some formulas can be stored in the refrigerator for up to 48 hours, while others must be used within 1 hour of mixing.

If your baby takes only part of her bottle and you think she may take more, you may feed her the remainder of her bottle within 1 hour of the beginning of the feeding. After this, used formula should be discarded because it is a breeding ground for bacteria. If the formula you choose is one that can be prepared in advance, you can carry it with you in its prepared state. Once it has been out of the refrigerator for more than 1 hour, it should be disposed of.

DID YOU KNOW?

EXPIRED FORMULA

Cans of formula (liquid and powdered) have expiry dates. Never use formula that has expired. Most formula companies recommend using up a can of powdered formula within 1 month after it is opened. After that, the remaining contents should be discarded.

Feeding Schedule

Many parents wonder how much formula they should feed their baby, and how often. They worry they are feeding too much or too little, and aren't sure how to tell when their child is satisfied and when she is still hungry.

Full Babies

Babies indicate they are full by falling asleep, by playing with the nipple of the bottle (for example, chewing on it), by stopping sucking, by crying when you try to give them the bottle, or by turning their head away from the bottle.

Never force your baby to eat more once she has indicated that she is full. Even if she takes only 2 ounces (60 mL) of a 4-ounce (120 mL) bottle, resist the urge to try to get her to finish the whole bottle. On the other hand, if your baby still seems hungry after finishing a bottle, give her more.

Babies go through many growth changes, and their feeding habits change regularly. A baby knows how much she wants and how often, and she will tell you as much — you just need to learn how to read her cues.

Formula-Feeding Schedule

The table that follows is a convenient guide to how much and how often to feed your baby in the first year. Remember, some babies will eat more and some will eat less, so expect deviations from this schedule. If you are concerned that your baby is not taking enough formula, you will need to assess her output from her urine and stool patterns, as well as her weight, which your health-care provider can best evaluate. In the first few months, babies generally gain ⅔ to 1 ounce (20 to 30 grams) a day.

Recommended Feeding Schedule for Formula-Fed Babies

AGE	FEEDINGS PER DAY	AMOUNT PER FEED
0–1 week	6–10	2–3 oz (60–90 mL)
1–4 weeks	6–8	3–4 oz (90–120 mL)
1–3 months	5–6	4–6 oz (120–180 mL)
3–7 months	4–5	6–7 oz (180–210 mL)
7–12 months	3–4	7–8 oz (210–240 mL)

Adapted with permission from Daina Kalnins and Joanne Saab, *Better Baby Food, Second Edition* (Toronto: Robert Rose, 2008).

Managing Bottle-Feeding Problems

Parents sometimes run into problems with getting their babies to take a bottle. In some cases, the problems arise when a mother who has been breast-feeding tries to feed her baby formula from a bottle or when another caregiver tries to give a bottle of formula. Parents may fear that they will never be able to leave their child with a caregiver and spend time alone. At times, a baby who has always been bottle-fed may also refuse a bottle. These two different situations need to be treated differently.

Breast-Fed Babies

If your baby has been breast-fed before being introduced to formula in a bottle, there are different ways to prevent her from refusing the bottle:

- Once breast-feeding is well established, try giving your baby a bottle of expressed breast milk on a regular basis to ease the transition.

HOW TO: Feed Your Baby with a Bottle

1. Before feeding your baby a bottle, be sure the formula is mixed well, especially if you are using powdered formula. Otherwise, it may clog the nipple, and your baby may seem like she doesn't want the bottle when, in reality, she can't get any formula out of the nipple. Also make sure the nipple size is appropriate, so that the formula drips out easily.
2. Find a comfortable place for both of you. Sitting in a chair or sofa, cradle your baby's head in your arm. You may want to put a pillow under your arm or under your baby for support.
3. Position your baby so that her head is aligned with but slightly higher than the rest of her body. Never lay a baby flat to feed: because of the angle of the inner ear canal, if a baby is lying flat, formula could potentially flow into her ear when she swallows. Formula can act as a breeding ground for bacteria, leading to ear infections.
4. Next, take the nipple and stroke it along your baby's cheek. This should cause your baby to turn toward the bottle and open her mouth. If she is asleep, you will need to wake her up before you do this. Once she opens her mouth, insert the bottle for her to feed.
5. Make sure that you always hold the bottle. Never prop it up with a towel or cloth: this can be very dangerous for your baby, as small babies cannot remove a bottle if they are choking on formula.
6. When you hold the bottle, make sure the nipple is filled with formula at all times to prevent your baby from sucking in air, which can cause discomfort.
7. Look into your baby's eyes when she is feeding, and talk or sing to her. This is your special time with your baby — enjoy every minute.

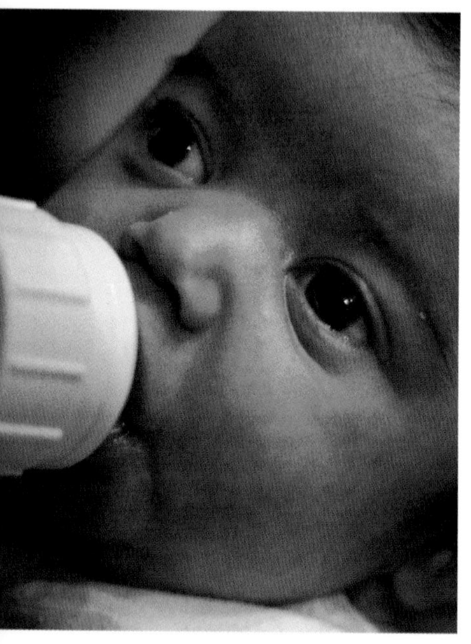

- Check to be sure you have an appropriate nipple. The solution may be as simple as changing nipples.
- Try having someone else offer your baby the bottle, preferably while you are out of the room. Because most babies prefer to breast-feed, they may not take the bottle from their mother.
- Try offering breast milk in the bottle instead of formula. If this is not successful, switch to formula.

If your baby still refuses the bottle (which is quite possible), you may have to wait until she is hungry enough. A hungry baby will feed eventually, even from a bottle she previously refused.

Bottle-Fed Babies

If your baby has always been bottle-fed and is now refusing the bottle, here is some advice:

- Make sure there is nothing wrong with the bottle or the formula (for example, expired formula or blocked nipple).
- Do not change formulas abruptly without advice from your child's health-care provider. The formula is usually not the issue.
- Remember that a baby's eating habits change as she grows, and her appetite may suddenly increase or decrease. If your child is taking less formula but her urine and stool patterns are the same, this eating pattern may be the new normal for her.
- If your baby is refusing to eat altogether, ask your health-care provider to assess your baby's health.

KEY POINT

Never force your baby to take a bottle. This could result in a feeding aversion.

Burping Your Baby

Whether you choose to breast-feed or formula-feed your baby, she may need to be burped as part of her feeding routine. The air babies swallow collects in their tummies, creating increased pressure and subsequent discomfort. Burping allows this air to be released, relieving discomfort and creating room for more milk. Some babies require burping during the feeding (stop feeding, burp, then resume), while others can wait until the end.

Different babies require different amounts of burping. Not all babies burp at every feeding. There are no strict rules for exactly when they should burp. With practice, you will come to know what works for your baby. For more information, see How to Burp Your Baby (page 84).

DID YOU KNOW?

SPITTING UP

Many babies spit up after a feeding, so don't be alarmed if your baby does. Properly burping her may decrease the chances that she will spit up.

Spitting Up

Most infants regurgitate milk or formula from the stomach through the mouth or nose. Do not be alarmed: this is a normal event. In babies, the esophagus (the feeding tube that connects the mouth to the stomach) is relatively small, and the muscle at the end is not always fully developed. The result is gastroesophageal reflux — more commonly called spitting up. This is different from forceful vomiting; it's an effortless regurgitation from the stomach back into the esophagus.

HOW TO: Burp Your Baby

If you are breast-feeding, burp your baby immediately after she finishes feeding on one breast. If she feeds on both breasts during a feeding, she will need to be burped twice. If you are bottle-feeding, you may need to interrupt the feeding halfway through to burp your baby.

The techniques for burping are the same for breast-fed and bottle-fed babies. A successful technique requires that you apply mild pressure to the baby's abdomen and hold her head elevated above her stomach. Some babies will even burp on their own when brought from a lying to an upright position. You can use one of the following three techniques, or you may find another one that is comfortable for you and your baby.

1. Hold your baby in an upright position with her arms over your shoulder and her tummy resting on your shoulder. Gently rub or pat her back.
2. Hold your baby in a seated position on your lap. With one hand, support her jaw using your thumb and index finger while applying pressure to her abdomen with the heel of that same hand. Gently pat or rub her back with the other hand.
3. Hold your baby so that she is lying stomach down in your lap with her legs hanging off one side. Support her head by holding her chin with your index finger and thumb. Gently rub or pat her back with the other hand.

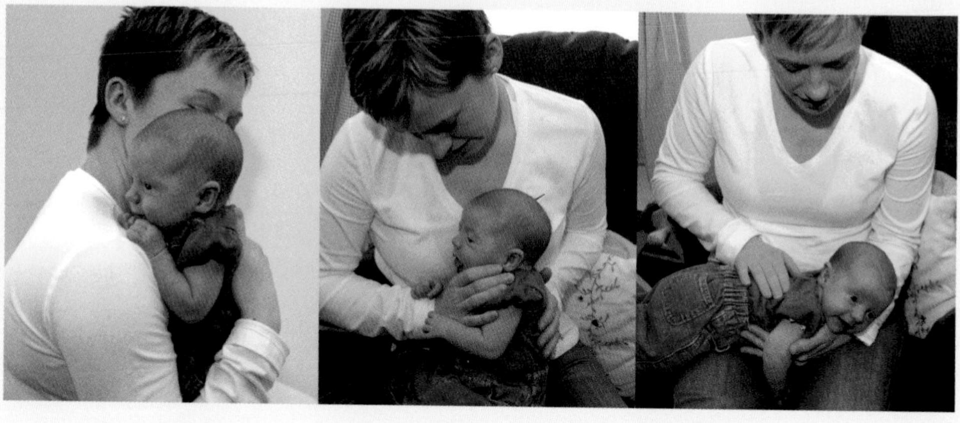

Reflux Facts

For most babies, reflux is not bothersome — but parents can be surprised by its impact on the laundry pile! If the milk made its way to the stomach before coming back up, it may have curdled and will smell sour, but otherwise the contents will be just like the milk your baby was fed.

Like most things, there is much variation in how often each baby spits up. Some do so only occasionally, while others spit up many times each day.

Spitting up does not interfere with feeding or growth and should be considered a normal part of infancy. The reality is, if your baby is a "spitter," there is little you will be able to do to change this! Rest assured that it will come to an end. Spitting up is most common in the first few months; it improves spontaneously and becomes an infrequent occurrence (less than 5% of infants) by 1 year of age. Many parents find that it settles down when their baby begins to sit upright or starts on solid foods.

When to Be Concerned

A minority of infants do have significant problems that can be related to reflux, including poor weight gain, discomfort during feeding, blood loss from the digestive tract due to the irritation of stomach acid, or recurrent respiratory problems (gagging, cough, or pneumonia) due to aspiration.

Reflux Red Flags

If you notice any of these red flags, consult with your baby's doctor:

- Your baby is not gaining weight.
- She is arching with feeds.
- She is refusing to feed.
- She is gagging or coughing persistently.
- She is vomiting forcefully.
- The spit-up contains tiny bits of blood or pieces of digested blood that resemble coffee grounds.
- The spit-up is dark green (bilious) in color.

Spitting-Up Strategies

Though there is no cure for simple spitting up, you may find these strategies helpful:

- Avoid overstimulating your baby following her feeds.
- Burp her in the middle of each feed as well as at the end.
- If you're bottle-feeding, ensure that the bottle is tilted up to minimize the amount of air in the nipple.
- Stay as dry as possible by keeping a burping cloth over your shoulder, carry a change of clothes for your baby when you go out, and stock up on laundry detergent!

DID YOU KNOW?

THRIVING

To parents, the quantity of regurgitated milk often makes it look as though the whole feed has come back up. The reality is that much less is actually regurgitated. Despite appearances, the majority of babies who spit up are keeping down all the milk they need, and the amount that is regurgitated is relatively insignificant. The ultimate test is whether your baby is gaining weight. If she is feeding well and thriving, her spitting up is an annoyance but not a concern, even if it looks like nothing is staying down.

KEY POINT

Every parent should be prepared with knowledge of infant CPR. Ask your local hospital or public health unit for available courses.

DID YOU KNOW?

RECOMMENDED DOSAGE

The current recommendation by the American Academy of Pediatrics and the Canadian Paediatric Society is that breast-fed babies be given a vitamin D supplement starting shortly after birth. Formulas are fortified with vitamin D. Children who are partially breast-fed and receive supplemental formula may not require extra vitamin D, provided they drink over 34 ounces (1,000 mL) of formula a day. In the United States and Canada, the recommended dose of vitamin D is 400 IU (international units) a day. In Canada, the recommended dose in very northern communities is 800 IU a day.

Gagging and Choking

Once an infant's feeding is established, it is normal for her to occasionally choke on breast milk or formula after taking a big gulp. This is particularly true if you are nursing and have a fast letdown reflex or if your baby spits up and chokes on the regurgitated milk. When this happens, lean your baby forward or over your shoulder, gently rub her back, and allow her to cough and catch her breath.

If your baby is choking and is unable to clear her own airway, call for an ambulance immediately. If necessary, and if you know how, initiate infant CPR.

Nutrient Supplements

Whether you choose to breast-feed or formula-feed your baby, at some point in the first year she will require nutrient supplements, specifically vitamin D, iron, and perhaps fluoride.

Vitamin D

Children need vitamin D to build strong bones. If they don't get enough vitamin D, infants are at risk of developing rickets, a disease that causes the bones to become soft, weak, and subsequently deformed.

There are several sources of vitamin D. Some foods, such as salmon, contain it, and cow's milk is often fortified with it. The skin can also produce vitamin D when it is exposed to sunlight. People with darker skin require more sunlight exposure to create the same amount of vitamin D as people with lighter skin.

Children at greatest risk of getting rickets are those who live in colder climates, where they may not be exposed to enough direct sunlight. This is especially true for children with darker skin, particularly if their mother has a vitamin D deficiency or if they are exclusively breast-fed. Breast milk contains vitamin D, but only in minute quantities.

Exposing children to sunlight is one way to ensure that they get enough vitamin D, but this is not always practical and carries the long-term risk of skin cancer. Sunscreen prevents the skin from making vitamin D. Therefore, leading pediatric health-care agencies recommend that all babies take vitamin D in supplemental form.

Iron

Babies are typically born with good iron reserves, received from their mothers during pregnancy. When these reserves are combined with the iron provided by breast milk, most babies have enough iron in their diet until they are 6 months of age. However, if iron-containing solid foods or iron-fortified formula and cereals are not introduced at that time, your baby could become iron-deficient, resulting in anemia, irritability, and decreased activity. Iron deficiency may also adversely affect development.

Fluoride

Fluoride is important for the development of healthy teeth. Children may require supplemental fluoride if their water supply contains less than 0.3 ppm (mcg per L). Check with your municipality to see if your tap water is fluoridated and consult with your baby's health-care provider to discuss whether supplementation is advisable.

DID YOU KNOW?

SOURCES OF IRON

Meat, green vegetables, and iron-fortified cereals are all high in iron. In general, if these are introduced to your baby's diet when she is around 6 months of age, no further iron supplements will be required.

GUIDE TO: Supplemental Fluids

Children under 1 year of age do not need to drink any fluids besides formula or breast milk and water. Although many companies sell juice for infants — advertising its vitamin C content, for example — your baby does not need it. Vitamin C is also present in breast milk and formula, which are much more complete sources of nutrition. The healthiest option is to avoid giving your baby juice in the first year.

Supplemental Water

Formula will generally provide all the water an infant needs. Extra water is seldom necessary. Still, when it is very hot outside, formula-fed infants can be given supplemental water.

Babies who are breast-fed do not require extra water. A mother's milk contains approximately 88% water, which is enough fluid to satisfy the baby. Even in hot climates, allowing your baby to have as many extra feeds as she wants will be sufficient to ensure adequate hydration.

Supplemental Formula

Babies who are breast-fed and who are growing well do not need supplemental formula. Breast milk provides all the calories and protein a baby requires in the first 6 months. However, supplementation may be appropriate if your baby's weight gain is poor. If you are concerned about your baby's growth, discuss it with your health-care provider. The goal should always be to ensure a healthy, thriving baby.

Frequently Asked Questions

My 5-month-old daughter has been solely breast-fed, yet this week she came down with a very bad cold and developed an ear infection. I thought breast-feeding was supposed to prevent her from getting sick. What happened?

There is no doubt that breast-feeding provides your baby with protective antibodies that measurably reduce the chances of various infections, such as gastroenteritis, colds, and serious blood-borne illnesses. Unfortunately, breast-feeding does not guarantee complete protection for all the common infections of childhood. Breast-fed babies will still get sick sometimes. In fact, they need exposure to the common viruses to stimulate their immune systems.

I considered my options carefully and chose to formula-feed my baby because of personal circumstances. Maybe it's my own guilt that is troubling me, but I can't help feeling that my friends, my relatives, and even my colleagues disapprove of my choice. Did I make a mistake?

No one but you walks in your shoes. Without thorough knowledge of your situation, no one has the right to judge you. Yet, it is very easy for a vulnerable individual to be upset by the opinionated and judgmental. Although breast-feeding has definite advantages and is recommended as the preferred form of infant nutrition, there are practical reasons that might preclude it as an option. You considered your options carefully, so trust yourself and your decision. If you remain troubled, discuss your feelings with your health-care provider.

Some authorities recommend scheduled feedings for young breast-fed infants, while others advise feeding on demand. Which should I choose?

Some parents, especially first-time mothers and fathers, need structure and routine to feel confident in their parenting skills. Others are comfortable recognizing their baby's cues and prefer to feed on demand. No single method is superior, so choose what works best for you. In practice, there isn't much difference between the feeding methods. Young infants naturally feed 8 to 12 times a day, which is what they tend to get by routine or by demand. Besides, few mothers will let a hungry baby continue to cry without feeding her, even if it is earlier than her schedule suggests.

When should a cup be introduced?

There is no rush; wait until your baby can sit supported. Drinking from a cup in the sitting position reduces the risk of choking, compared to drinking while supine (on the back). Babies at 4 to 6 months of age are quite "oral": they love to explore with their mouths. If you are interested in supplementing breast-feedings, it is quite reasonable to introduce a cup at this age.

CHAPTER 4

Your Baby's First Month

Congratulations! By now, you have mastered the important skills of holding, bathing, dressing, and feeding your baby. Don't underestimate your achievement. You are back at home and likely in the process of moving on from the chaotic first few days following your baby's birth and establishing routines. The first few weeks of your baby's life are a time for settling in, getting to know your baby, and adjusting to your new family.

As the initial crowds of visitors start to thin a bit, and your energy starts to wane, you may be starting to think about what life with your baby is going to be like. What will you do all day? Will you have a schedule or routine? For goal-oriented parents, routines may give a sense of accomplishment at the end of the day.

In the first month of life, you should not expect your newborn to display the regularity of a clock, feeding every 3 hours or sleeping precisely every 2 hours. Most babies will eat, then sleep, then have quiet awake time. The amount of time in each of these periods will vary. You may want to use that sleep interval to catch up on your own sleep or do some necessary household activities. Also try to take even a few minutes for yourself. You could spend your baby's awake period reading to him, showing him objects and shapes, listening to music, or taking him for a walk. This approach breaks up your day (and night) into manageable segments.

DID YOU KNOW?

A TRANSITIONAL STAGE

The first month of your baby's life is a sharp transitional stage. Prior to delivering your baby, you may have held down a job and been involved in sports, with an active social life. You had plenty of time to do the things that you wanted to do. This is still achievable, but probably not in the first month. This time is all about getting to know your baby and discovering what works best for him and for you.

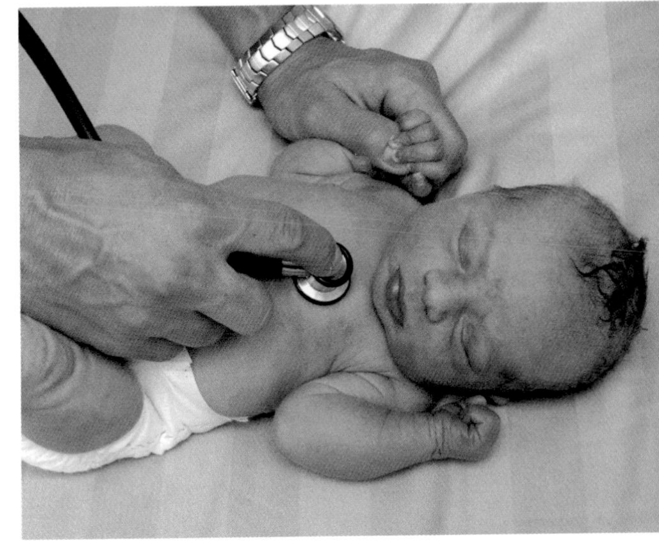

First Visit to Your Baby's Doctor

Part of your routine will be regular visits to your baby's doctor. The first visit is usually within a few days of your baby being discharged from the hospital. This early follow-up visit enables prompt detection of significant feeding issues, dehydration, or excessive jaundice.

This will be the first of many health maintenance visits for you and your baby, designed to address any concerns or questions you have, review your baby's growth parameters and developmental milestones, discuss age-related safety tips, examine your child from head to toe, and provide immunizations, if needed. During these visits, you and your doctor will get to know one another. The doctor-parent relationship is very important.

GUIDE TO: Visiting Your Baby's Doctor

There are some things you can do to make the most of your regular visits to your baby's doctor, starting with the first visit in the first month:

- Ideally, both parents should attend these visits. If only one parent can attend, try to have a friend or trusted relative accompany you to help with the baby so you can concentrate on the discussion at hand. This may be the first time you have left home with your baby, and an extra adult can be very helpful, if only to carry the diaper bag and hold open the doors.
- Some parents like to prepare a written list of questions ahead of time. Otherwise, the minute you walk out of the office you're likely to remember all the questions you forgot to ask. Your doctor has a lot of experience in general child-care issues, parenting, and health promotion, but ask her to recommend additional resources if you feel you need further information.
- Most family doctors or pediatricians have busy waiting rooms; you may have to wait a while. Be prepared to amuse, comfort, and feed your baby while you wait.
- After going into an examining room, you will likely be asked by a nurse to undress your newborn. Your baby may first be weighed and measured by the nurse. Let the nurse know of any questions or concerns you have — nurses are often very experienced at dealing with these issues.
- Your doctor will likely inquire about your baby's feeding, sleeping, number of wet and dirty diapers, and how you as parents are coping with your newborn. Be prepared to answer these questions. The doctor may also ask about your own health and the health of your family, because some illnesses can run in families.
- The doctor will then examine your baby in detail from head to toe. Afterwards, you should have an opportunity to discuss any questions or concerns you have. Ensure that all of your questions are addressed and that you are comfortable with the answers. If you don't understand something, your doctor should be happy to review it with you or suggest an alternative source of information.
- Before you leave the office, make sure to learn the procedures for scheduling new appointments, whom to call after hours and on weekends with questions, and whether your doctor provides any telephone advice.

Growth During the First Month

From the moment your new arrival is placed on the scale, his growth will be the focus of much attention for you and your health-care provider. Your baby's weight, length, and head circumference will be measured at birth and before discharge from the hospital. Keep a record of these measurements and bring them to your child's checkups.

Infants grow and change rapidly throughout their first year. If you need any proof of this, just think about their constant need for new and bigger clothes! Adequate growth — in particular, weight gain — means that your baby is obtaining sufficient nutrition to support the amazing development he will undergo in the upcoming months.

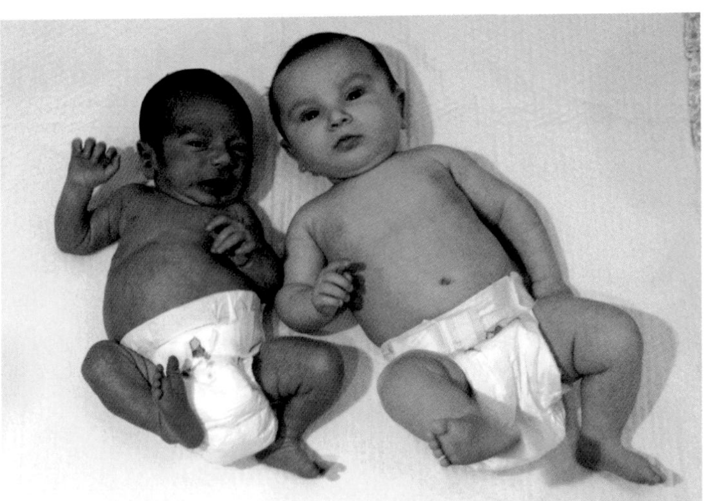

Measuring Your Baby

Health-care providers will periodically measure your baby's weight, length, and head circumference to ensure that he is growing normally. At every visit with your doctor, weight will be measured using an infant scale until your child is big enough to stand on a scale alone. An infant's length is most accurately measured using a special measurement board. A measuring tape wrapped around the largest part of the head (above the eyebrows and ears to the back of the head) is used to measure your baby's head circumference.

Weight Loss and Gain

Although growth and weight gain are important reflections of adequate nutrition, be aware that it is normal for your new baby to lose as much as 7% to 10% of his birth weight

KEY POINT

Your baby's weight will be followed closely throughout the newborn period. If weight loss is more than expected or is regained more slowly than usual, you will need to visit a doctor or clinic (for example, a breast-feeding clinic) more frequently to ensure that your baby is getting enough fluids and nutrition.

in the first few days of life. He should generally return to his birth weight within 10 days. Premature and smaller babies may require 2 weeks to return to their birth weight.

After this initial period of weight loss, if your baby is feeding well and is healthy, he will generally gain an average of $\frac{2}{3}$ to 1 ounce (20 to 30 g) every day. By the end of the first month, a baby who began life at a weight of 7.7 pounds (3.5 kg) will weigh about 10 pounds (4.5 kg). At 2 months, an average North American baby weighs between 9.5 and 15 pounds (4.4 and 7 kg).

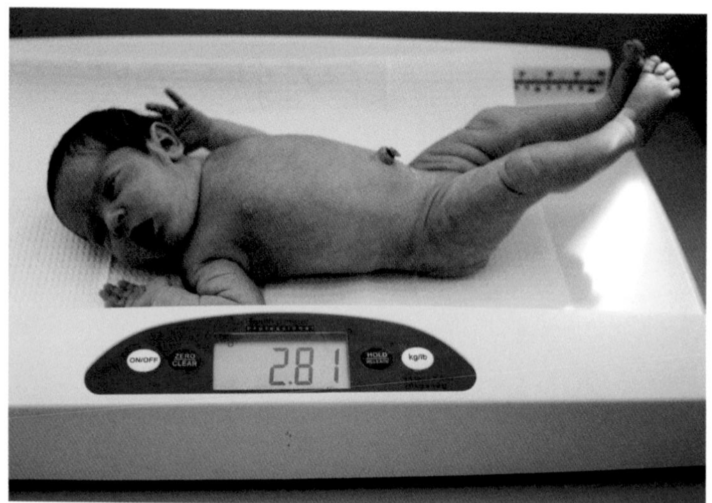

Length

Growth in length is slower than gain in weight. It is also more difficult to measure accurately. Your baby's length will be measured less frequently than his weight. During his first month, your baby will grow about 1.5 to 2 inches (4 to 5 cm). At 2 months, an average North American baby measures 21.5 to 24.5 inches (55 to 62 cm).

Head Circumference

Your child's head size is often a reflection of your own. If a baby's head measures larger than expected for her age, a doctor may measure both parents' heads to see whether they are also large. It is important that your child's head grows at the expected rate, following one of the curves on the growth chart. An infant's head usually grows 0.5 inch (1 cm) in diameter every 2 weeks for the first 3 months. If head growth is more rapid or slower than expected, medical tests may be recommended to determine the cause.

Growth Curves

Growth measurements are recorded on standard growth curves, which describe the range of normal weight, length, and head circumference for a given age and sex. There are separate growth curves for boys and girls, as girls tend to be smaller than boys and change in size at a slightly different rate. In North America, most health-care providers currently use growth curves developed by the World Health Organization. These can be found at: www.cdc.gov/growthcharts/who_charts.htm (U.S.) and www.whogrowthcharts.ca (Canada).

Reading the Curves

The 50th percentile on the growth curves describes the average weight, length, or head circumference measurement per age. The range of normal measurements falls between the 3rd and the 97th percentiles. For example, the average weight for a newborn baby born within 2 weeks of the expected due date is 7.25 pounds (3.3 kg), average height is 19.5 inches (50 cm), and average head circumference is 14 inches (35 cm). However, any weight between 5.5 and 9 pounds (2.5 and 4 kg) would be considered within the normal range. Similarly, birth length between 18 and 21 inches (46 and 53 cm) is considered appropriate.

By plotting growth measurements on a growth curve, your doctor will determine whether they fall within the typical range, whether your baby is growing proportionately (his weight is appropriate for his length), and whether he is growing at the expected rate (typically following one of the curves).

Deviations from these expectations may mean that your child is simply expressing his own unique growth pattern. However, poor growth can sometimes indicate a problem, such as insufficient nutrition or a medical disorder. Such a finding may lead your doctor to recommend adjustments to feeding or to do some tests to look for a medical explanation while following your baby's growth more closely.

DID YOU KNOW?

SIZE AT BIRTH

Just like adults, babies are quite different from one another. Some begin life smaller, some larger, some leaner, and some chubbier. A baby's size at birth may be affected by his mother's health, nutrition, lifestyle, and weight gain during pregnancy, his parents' sizes, and blood flow through the placenta. Certain medical conditions during pregnancy, such as diabetes, may lead to a higher birth weight. Smoking, high blood pressure, health problems during pregnancy, or some medical problems in newborns may be associated with lower birth weights.

What will be most important over the upcoming months is the rate at which your child gains weight and grows.

Development During the First Month

During the first month of life, your baby will spend most of his time sleeping or feeding. Even though it may seem like that is all he is doing, he is developing a wider range of physical movements and reflexes, as well as exciting new communication behaviors.

What Newborns See

Newborn babies usually keep their eyes closed for the first few days of life. Your baby has emerged from the dark womb into a world filled with light and color.

Newborns can see most clearly at a distance of 8 to 10 inches (20 to 25 cm); this is also the usual distance from baby to mother's face during feeding. Studies have shown that newborns are drawn to the contrasting shapes and colors of a human face. They also like to look at pictures of faces and contrasting black and white geometrical shapes. Even babies under 1 month will try to focus on objects.

Babies' eyes, however, do not work together at this age, and crossed eyes are often the result. Crossed eyes should start to improve by 2 to 4 months of age as the baby's ability to use both eyes together (binocular vision) is established. Babies do not learn how to fixate and follow an object until 6 to 8 weeks of life.

When your baby is in a state of quiet alertness, hold him upright at 10 inches (25 cm) from your face and talk to him in a soft, high voice — he may respond and appear to be listening to and looking at you.

Physical Movements

Over the course of the month, you may notice some small increases in your baby's quiet awake time. His arms and legs, which are initially held bent up toward his body, will relax soon after birth. He may begin to organize his jerky wiggles into more organized movements and pauses. An infant of this age has very limited ability to hold up his relatively large head with his developing neck muscles and still requires your gentle support.

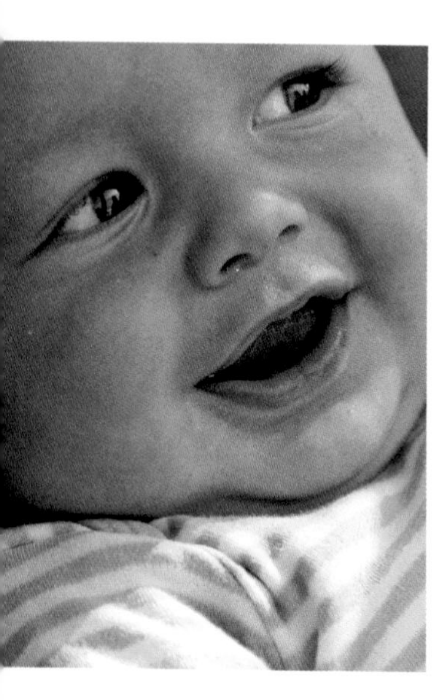

Smiling

As the first month progresses, an infant starts to pay attention to caregivers' faces, watching and following them with his eyes. Infants at this age cannot see details well, but do notice large mouth movements, such as your big smile! Your baby now tends to settle when picked up and watches your face intently when being spoken to or fed. It is heartwarming to see your baby's smiles, even though they are initially a "reflex." But very soon they should start to become purposeful and responsive, usually by 6 weeks of age. This is one of the first milestones that many health-care professionals will inquire about.

Communication

Your baby will appear to look around and may respond to noises. This is the time when you and your baby learn to communicate with each other. Your baby is learning to trust you. Your responses to his crying — picking him up, comforting him, and providing him with food, a diaper change, or warmth — all contribute to this growing bond. You cannot spoil your baby at this age.

Your baby will communicate with you throughout this period mainly by crying and cooing. "Cooing" refers to the "aaah" sounds young infants make; they make your sleepless nights seem worthwhile. If you respond to these noises by imitating them softly, it will help your baby develop early language skills.

DID YOU KNOW?

SOOTHING SOUNDS

Babies' hearing is fully developed at birth. They often prefer high-pitched voices, and studies have shown that some babies are soothed by familiar sounds they were exposed to during your pregnancy. You don't need to tiptoe around your baby, but babies do not like overstimulation. A safe rule of thumb is to play music at a level you can comfortably talk over.

Development Milestones

Your baby's development will follow a relatively predictable pattern. The achievement of the common developmental milestones usually follows a recognizable sequence, but you must remember that the exact rate will vary a lot from child to child. If you expect your little champ to meet every milestone at the same time as, or even before, his peers in your mothers' group, then you are setting yourself up for unnecessary anxiety and disappointment.

Just like a child's growth patterns, the progression of a baby's development over time is what is most important. We know that some babies will walk at 9 months and others at 15 months, just as some will grow on the 10th percentile and others will grow on the 90th percentile curve. Developmental variations do not necessarily indicate that one child is "smarter" or more athletic than another. Even siblings can vary in when they start to walk or talk ... or show their temperament.

KEY POINT

Reading to your baby, even from a very early age, has been shown to have a positive effect on his cognitive development.

Advancing Development

There really isn't much that has been shown to increase the rate of a child's development, beyond what most parents do instinctively. Playing with your child, caring for him,

Development Milestones, First Year

AGE	GROSS MOTOR SKILLS *(How Your Baby Moves)*	FINE MOTOR SKILLS *(How Your Baby Uses His Hands)*	LANGUAGE	SOCIAL DEVELOPMENT AND PLAY
1 month	• Wiggles • Moves arms and legs • Stretches out arms and legs when startled • Has little control of head — flops around if unsupported	• Holds hands closed most of the time	• Crying • Cooing ("aah" sounds)	• Looks at caregiver's face
2 to 3 months	• Kicks legs • Supports head briefly when held upright • Is able to lift head briefly when placed on tummy	• Holds hands open most of the time	• Crying • Cooing	• Quiets when caregiver talks • Smiles responsively by 6 weeks • Looks toward sound • Follows moving object 180 degrees
4 to 6 months	• Turns around when lying on stomach • Rolls over, initially stomach to back and then back to stomach • Has good head control when pulled to sitting from lying or held upright • Lifts head and shoulders when placed on tummy	• Reaches for objects • Holds objects in hands and begins to transfer them from one hand to the other	• Cooing in imitation and response to adult sounds • Babbling and squealing • Razzing sounds ("raspberries")	• Bats at objects • Laughs • Is interested in own image in mirror • Puts toys in mouth • Becomes wary of strangers

AGE	GROSS MOTOR SKILLS *(How Your Baby Moves)*	FINE MOTOR SKILLS *(How Your Baby Uses His Hands)*	LANGUAGE	SOCIAL DEVELOPMENT AND PLAY
7 to 9 months	• Sits unsupported • Crawls • May pull to standing position	• Holds objects and bangs them • Starts to pick up small objects • Can feed himself a cracker	• Babbling (ba-ba-ba, da-da-da)	• Looks for toys that fall or roll out of sight • Plays peekaboo • Is reluctant to go to strangers
10 to 12 months	• Pulls to standing position • Walks along furniture (cruising) or with hand held • May start to walk independently (12 to 15 months)	• Holds cup • Picks up small objects • Points • Holds crayon in fist (12 months) • Puts small objects in container	• First words with meaning (12 months), usually "mama" or "dada" • Imitates speech	• Claps hands • Plays patty-cake • Waves "bye-bye" • Rolls a ball • Removes socks

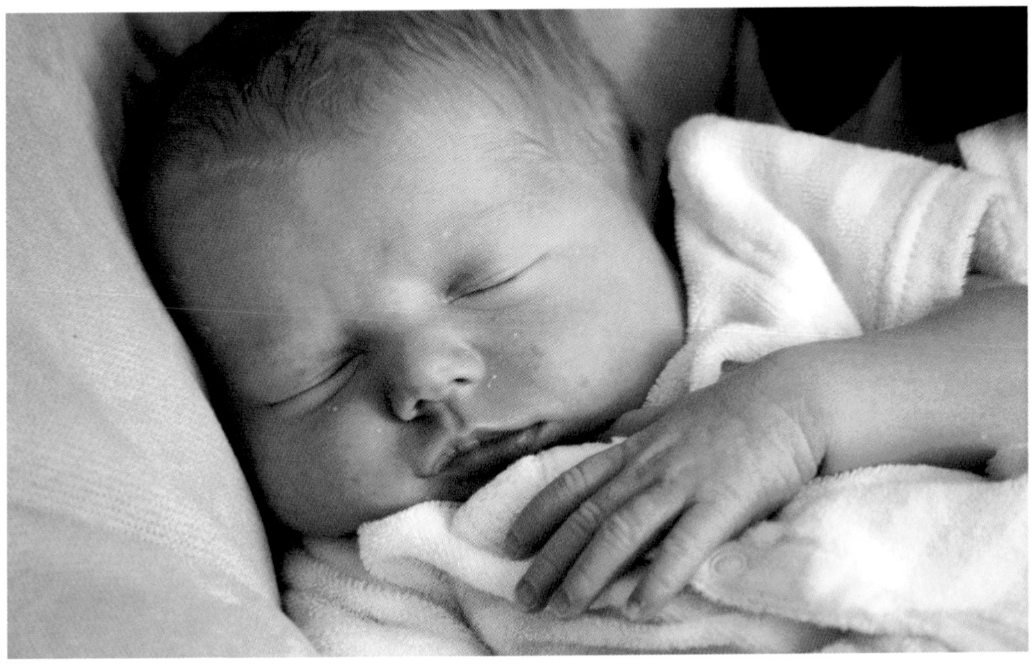

stimulating him, talking, reading, and singing to him, and, of course, loving him is how you can best help him reach his full potential.

Developmental Delay

If your child's development falls outside of the typical ranges in the table above, it may reflect a variation of normal or may indicate a problem that needs assessment and intervention. If your child's development plateaus so that he is not progressing over the course of months, or if his development actually regresses and he loses some of his previous skills, he should be carefully assessed by your health-care provider.

Trust your instincts if you are concerned in any way about your child's development, and be sure to mention this to your doctor. Despite the wide variation in normal, a parent's intuition is very important. If you suspect your child may be experiencing a developmental delay, consult with your child's health-care provider.

Warning Signs of Possible Developmental Delay

AREA OF DEVELOPMENT	WARNING SIGN
Gross motor development	• Rolling prior to 3 months • Not walking by 18 months
Fine motor development	• Holding hands tightly in fists for most of the time at 3 months • Preferring left or right hand before 18 months
Language development	• Not pointing by 12 months • Not using three words by 15 months • Not turning when name is called at 18 months • Not able to identify body parts by 2 years
Social development	• Not interested in other children at 2 years • No imaginary play at 2 years

Irregular and Noisy Breathing

If you watch your baby breathe, you will notice that he takes many short breaths of different lengths, the occasional deep breath and sigh, and even pauses of 8 to 10 seconds between breaths. This irregular breathing pattern, called periodic breathing, is normal; breathing usually becomes more regular around the end of the first month of life.

Many babies also breathe noisily, which many mistake for a cold or congestion. A newborn's nasal passages are very small, and even a slight amount of blockage can cause noisy breathing. Your baby may appear to be struggling to breathe through his nose and may sneeze to clear his passages. Frequent sneezing is not a sign that he has a cold, but rather a protective reflex to clear his nose.

Here are a few strategies to clear your baby's nose:

- To decrease irritation, lessen your baby's exposure to environmental irritants such as dust, lint, and tobacco smoke.
- If the nasal congestion seems to be interfering with feeding or sleeping, try nasal drops or a suction bulb, but only continue if it seems to be helping. Theoretically, saline or salt water nose sprays or drops can loosen up the nasal mucus, allowing it to drain more freely or making it easier to suck out with a nasal aspirator. However, the use of nasal drops or aspirators has not been well studied for this purpose; they are often felt to be ineffective.

KEY POINT

If your baby has a sudden onset of noisy breathing or changes in his breathing pattern, or if his breathing seems labored or difficult, it is best to see your doctor.

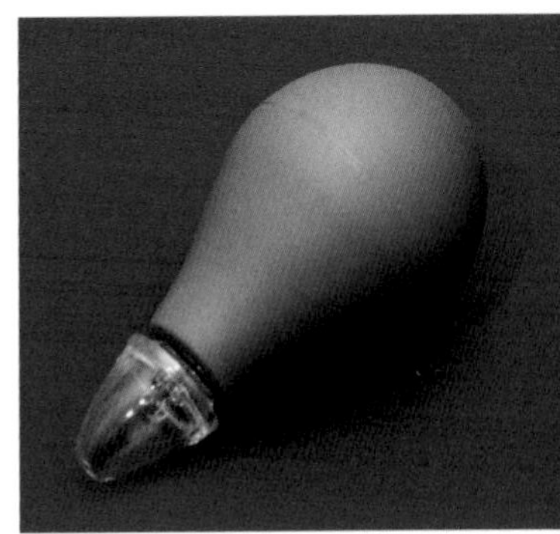

Interpreting Crying

Babies cry to communicate what they need because they can do little for themselves. As your baby gets older, he will learn to use other sounds, facial expressions, and gestures to communicate his needs. Realistically, however, he will continue to cry from time to time.

As parents, we are often sleep-deprived and worried, which makes interpretation very challenging at times. Use these questions to try to identify why your baby might be crying:

1. **Are you hungry?** Most babies will cry when they are hungry. Your baby may put his hand to his mouth, suck vigorously on a finger or pacifier, smack his lips, or root. Try offering your baby a feed.
2. **Do you need a diaper change?** Babies vary in how long they will tolerate a wet or soiled diaper. Some will want to be changed right away; others don't seem to notice. A clean diaper will quickly resolve crying as a result of a dirty bottom.

KEY POINT

Not all crying means that your baby is hungry. Consider other possibilities.

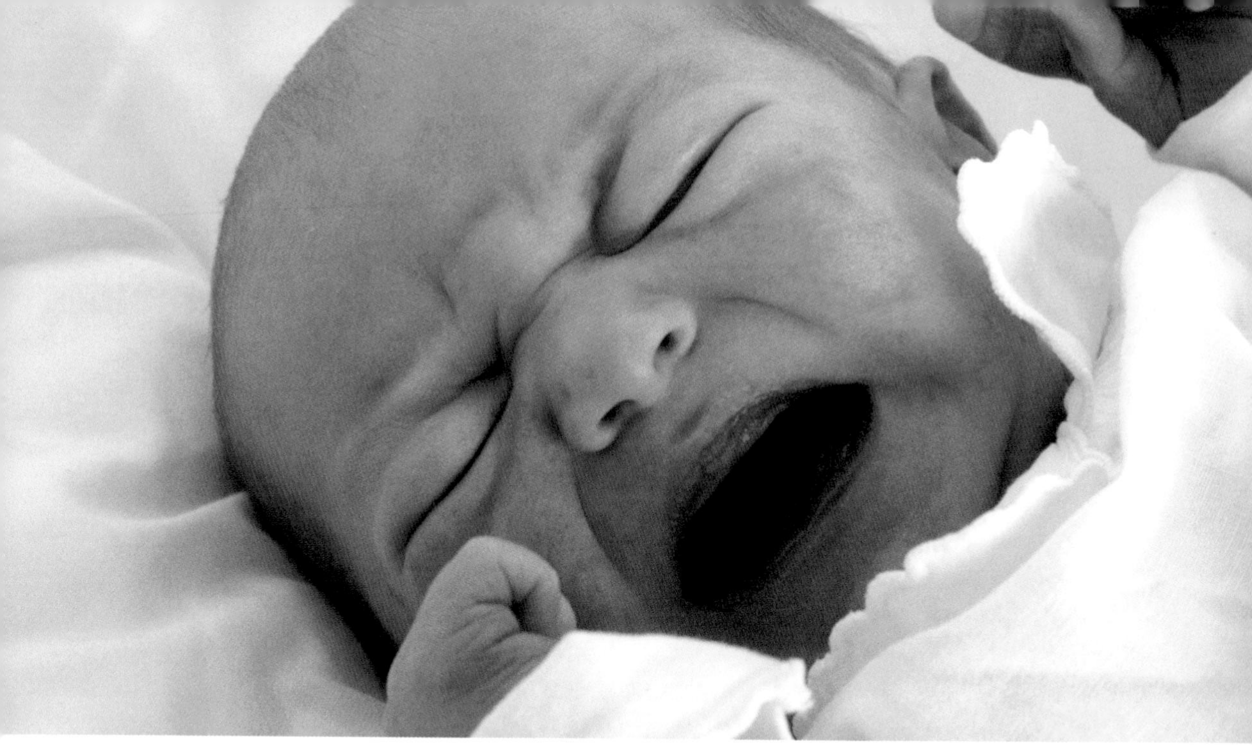

3. **Are you tired?** Babies need a lot of rest, but often have difficulty soothing themselves to sleep. They will often fuss, cry, and become agitated or inconsolable when they need to sleep, especially if they are overtired. A young baby may need your help falling asleep; removing stimulation and providing a calm, dark, and quiet environment may help. Some babies may also need to be rocked, swaddled, or otherwise soothed to sleep.
4. **Do you want to be held?** Babies love to be held close in order to feel, hear, and smell their caregivers. Many people worry about spoiling a baby by carrying them too much, but you cannot spoil a baby with attention in the first few months of life. If your baby wants to be held all the time, you may find an infant carrier helpful and convenient.
5. **Is your tummy bothering you?** Gas can make an infant uncomfortable. Infants may pull up their legs, pass gas, or strain and grunt when passing stool. Try placing your baby on his belly, moving his legs back and forth in a bicycling motion, or giving him a gentle tummy massage. There are many over-the-counter medications for gas. They have not been scientifically proven to work, but, on the other hand, they are generally not harmful. If you suspect gas is the source of your baby's crying, discuss these options with your health-care provider.

6. **Do you need to burp?** Crying that occurs during or after a feed can be due to gas or liquid and stomach acid traveling back up the esophagus. Babies can swallow a lot of air while breast- or bottle-feeding and may need to burp during or after feeding. Some babies burp spontaneously, but others need help to do so. See page 84 for burping techniques.
7. **Are you too warm or cold?** Babies may feel too hot or too cold, and are very sensitive to being over- or underdressed. Generally, one light layer more than what an adult is wearing will keep a baby comfortable.
8. **Are you in pain?** Little things that can be hard to spot may be causing pain. Your baby may have a small cut or abrasion that is difficult to see, or a rough tag or stitching on clothing may be causing him discomfort. If you can't find any obvious reason for your baby's crying, undress him completely and give him a good once-over.
9. **Are you teething?** In general, the first tooth arrives between 6 and 10 months, but there is huge variation. A teething baby may drool or mouth objects more than usual. His gums may appear red or swollen, and you may be able to feel or see a hard white bump under the gums or breaking through. Teething pain may be relieved by over-the-counter pain medication, including acetaminophen, or by providing a cool, clean cloth or teething ring for your baby to chew on.
10. **Do you need stimulation or a break?** The sights, sounds, sensations, and smells of the world outside the womb are all new to a baby. Sometimes a baby may want to experience more of what is around him and he'll cry to tell you he needs more stimulation. Other times, a baby may cry to tell you there is too much going on and he needs a break. Finding the right amount of stimulation for your baby is a learning process, and that amount will change as your baby grows.
11. **Are you sick?** Babies may cry to tell you they are feeling sick. A sick baby may be less active, may not want to feed or may feed less, or may have a fever. Trust your instincts, because you know your baby best. If you suspect your baby is sick, talk to your doctor.

DID YOU KNOW?

CRYING TIME

Crying is perfectly normal, but there is a wide range of crying time. Some babies cry as little as 1 hour a day or less (lucky parents!), and others can cry for up to 5 or 6 hours a day. Crying increases over the first few weeks of life, reaching a peak at about 6 weeks.

Colic

Colic is usually defined as inconsolable crying, often in the evening, for at least 3 hours a day, at least 3 days a week, and at least 3 weeks in a row. During the episode, the baby may scream, turn red in the face, clench his fists, and pull up his legs.

There is much debate about the exact cause of colic. Some believe it is caused by gas, digestion problems, and abdominal pain. Others feel it is more a result of an immaturity of the nervous system and a difficulty regulating sensory information both from the environment and from within the body. Still others wonder if it is a manifestation of individual temperament or personality.

Regardless of the cause, no interventions have been shown to reliably treat colic. Babies suffering from colic can be very difficult to soothe, and will often cry no matter what you do. Thankfully, colic will resolve on its own, usually by 3 to 5 months of age.

HOW TO: Calm Your Colicky Baby

Colic can be very frustrating for parents. Try soothing your baby with these standard strategies for relief, but know that although some things will work some of the time, you may not find a technique that will work all of the time.

- **Swaddle:** Wrap your baby snugly in a warm blanket.
- **Sway:** Use rhythmic motion, such as swaying, swinging, bouncing, and vibration.
- **Stroll:** Take a walk with your baby in the stroller or drive him around in the car.
- **Pacify:** Give your baby a pacifier or a clean finger to suckle.
- **Calm:** Reduce stimulation by turning down the lights, reducing noise, or moving to a room alone with your baby.
- **Sing and play:** Play calming music, or sing, hum, or dance with your baby.
- **Create white noise:** Turn on a clothes dryer, vacuum cleaner, fan, faucet, or white noise machine.
- **Bathe:** Give your baby a warm bath or take a shower with him.
- **Go outside:** Bring your baby out into the fresh air — it may help him sleep.
- **Massage:** Slowly and gently rub your little one using baby lotion or oil.

If all these strategies fail, you may need to take a break. Put your baby in a safe place and take a minute for yourself. Call someone you trust for help. Talk about your frustration. Never, ever shake your baby.

Postpartum Blues

You have waited 9 months for your baby to arrive, feeling excitement, anticipation, and elation. Now that he has arrived, he seems to need you 24 hours a day. Your feelings may now be tinged with sadness, inadequacy, dread, and fear. In most cases, this is natural, but in some cases, these feelings can be more serious, leading to depression.

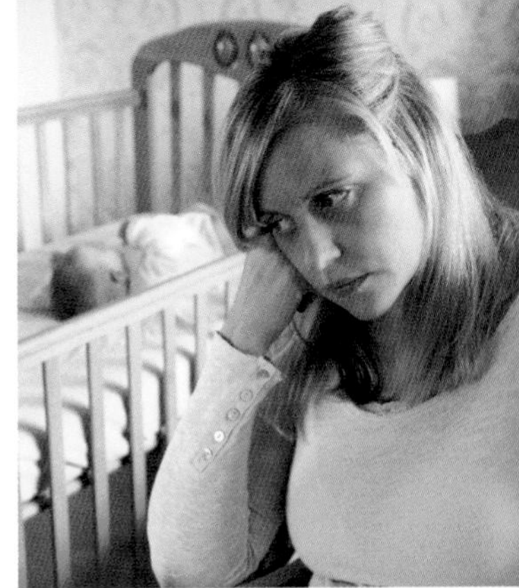

Baby Blues

Most new mothers have periods of weepiness, unhappiness, anxiety, and mood swings in the first week after delivery. Often called the baby blues, these feelings can be attributed to changes in hormone levels after delivery, changes in surroundings, and the new expectations of parenting. These feelings usually get better in 1 to 2 weeks and do not interfere with your ability to function.

Depression

About one in 10 women will have more severe symptoms of depression in the first year of her baby's life. Depression is a mood disorder in which feelings of sadness, loss, anger, or frustration interfere with everyday life for an extended period of time.

KEY POINT

Women with a previous history of depression or a family member with depression are at increased risk of postpartum depression, but most women with postpartum depression have no such history.

Symptoms of Postpartum Depression

Any of the following can be symptoms of depression if they last longer than 2 weeks:

- Feeling restless or irritable, sad, hopeless, or overwhelmed
- Crying often
- Lack of energy or motivation
- Eating too little or too much
- Sleeping too little or too much
- Trouble focusing, remembering, or making decisions
- Feeling worthless and guilty
- Loss of interest or pleasure in activities
- Withdrawal from friends and family
- Headaches, chest pains, heart palpitations (the heart beating fast and feeling like it is skipping beats), or hyperventilation (fast and shallow breathing)
- Fear of hurting the baby or yourself
- Lack of interest in the baby

Very rarely, symptoms can include delusions, hallucinations, or obsessive thoughts about the baby.

Treating Postpartum Depression

Some women keep their symptoms secret because they feel embarrassed, ashamed, or guilty about feeling depressed at a time when they are supposed to be happy. They worry they will be viewed as unfit parents. However, postpartum depression can happen to any woman. You and your baby don't have to suffer. There are effective treatments for depression and things you can try yourself:

KEY POINT

If you have symptoms of postpartum depression, know that you are not alone. Seek help from a medical professional for effective treatment strategies.

- Discuss these feelings with someone you trust, such as a family member, a friend, or your doctor.
- Try to get as much rest as you can; nap when the baby naps.
- Ask for help with household chores and nighttime feedings.
- Do not spend a lot of time alone. Get dressed and leave the house. Run an errand or take a short walk.
- Talk with other mothers, so you can learn from their experience.
- Seek medical treatment.

Getting Out of the House

Most new parents comment on how helpful it is to get out of the house. This may mean nothing more than a short walk, a visit to a friend, or a trip to the grocery store. If you feel up to it, go ahead and take your new baby out for a while.

The first expedition out of the house is a major step for new parents. Some need a U-Haul to cart around all their supplies. Others forget essentials, such as keys! It can all seem overwhelming at first, but soon enough you will have mastered the art of going outside.

KEY POINT

If strangers approach your baby and try to touch him (as they often do), don't feel embarrassed to say, "Please do not touch the baby. He bites!"

Where to Go

Wherever you choose to travel, avoid exposure to people with colds or obvious infections. Your new baby is at higher risk for complications from colds that seem minor in older children or adults. Don't take your newborn to a home with a child or adult who has cold or flu symptoms (fever, runny nose, cough, rash, diarrhea, or vomiting). You also may want to avoid large crowds. If you plan on going to a public place, do so in low-traffic times and in wide-open spaces.

When to Go

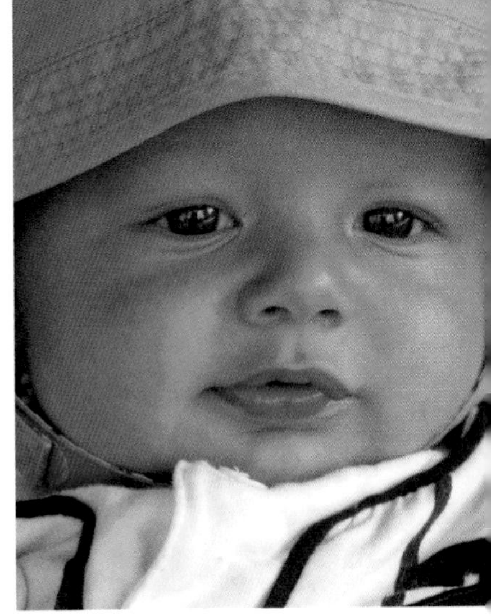

The timing of your outing is also important. You may want to plan it around your baby's schedule, such as after a feed. Make sure that you have the appropriate safety equipment ready, including an approved car seat, that he is properly buckled into his seat or stroller, and that he is adequately dressed for the weather. Babies can become hypothermic very quickly in winter, and they can sunburn easily in summer. On colder days, bundle your baby in as many layers as you would wear, plus an additional one, and protect him from wind, rain, and snow. In the summer, keep your baby shaded.

HOW TO: Dress Your Baby for Summer and Winter

Dressing your newborn baby during the first months can be frustrating – it sometimes seems as if you need a PhD in engineering to fasten all those snaps properly as your baby squirms. Dressing is further complicated when you live in a climate where the seasons change, requiring a whole new set of clothes and approach to dressing your baby. Like us, babies don't like to be too hot or too cold, regardless of the weather.

Summer Wear and Care

Being outdoors is very important for babies and parents, but make sure your baby is appropriately dressed for the weather and is protected from the sun and heat.

1. Don't overdress the baby so that he appears flushed, sweaty, or uncomfortable. A good rule of thumb for summer dressing is to dress him as you are dressed, then add one extra light layer.
2. Cool hands and feet may suggest that another layer of light clothing is needed.
3. Dress your baby in clothing that covers the body, such as comfortable lightweight long pants, long-sleeved shirts, and hats with brims that shade the face and cover the ears.
4. Babies younger than 6 months should be kept out of direct sunlight, so be sure to shade your child from the sun with a hat, screening umbrella, or stroller canopy. UV screens are available for strollers. When temperatures are very high (greater than 86°F/30°C) or there is a smog warning, limit your time outdoors. Sunscreen is not recommended at this young age because the risks and benefits of sunscreen use are not yet known. If your baby needs to be outdoors, discuss sunscreen use and other options with your health-care provider. Some authorities recommend zinc oxide or titanium dioxide, which are inert "sunblocks," for infants in the first

6 months if sun exposure cannot be prevented. If your baby gets a sunburn, see your doctor.

5. Do not leave your baby (or any child) alone in a car, even with the windows open. The inside of a car can heat up quickly to dangerous levels.
6. If your car has been parked outside on a hot day, make sure the car seat and seat belts are not hot before buckling your child into the car.

Winter Wear and Care

Infants are especially susceptible to fluctuations in external temperature because their bodies have a large surface area, allowing heat to be lost more easily through the head and skin, and because they cannot produce sufficient heat through shivering.

1. When you're going out in the cold, dress your infant in a number of layers. That way, articles of clothing can be easily removed or added as the weather dictates. A suitable outfit for an infant would include an undershirt, a sleeper, a snowsuit with coverings for hands and feet, a hat, and a blanket (not covering the face).
2. The extremities (hands and feet) and the lips, nose, and ears are the most susceptible to cold air and should be well protected.
3. When temperatures are very low (below −13°F/−25°C), keep your infant indoors or limit your time outdoors as much as possible. Seek medical attention immediately if your baby's skin becomes pale or blistered (signs of frostbite), if your baby becomes very sleepy and difficult to rouse, or if he becomes cold to the touch (signs of hypothermia).

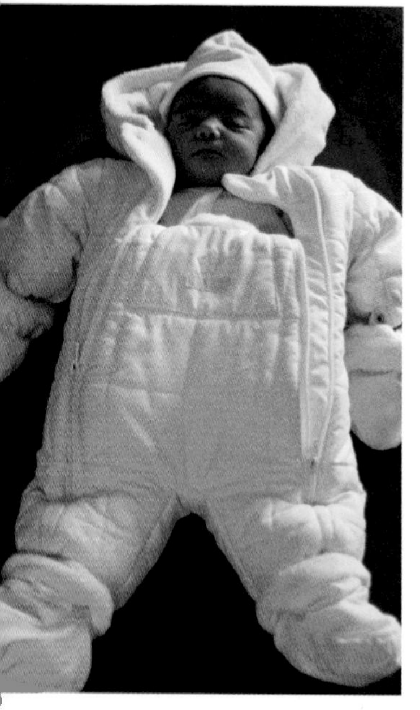

Receiving Visitors

In the first month of your baby's life, you will be reeling from sleep deprivation, will feel constantly rushed, and will not always look your best. This is not a great time to entertain every relative, friend, neighbor, and casual acquaintance who wants to meet your baby. You may be excited to show off your beautiful newborn, but a constant stream of people into your home is likely not good for you or your baby.

Here are some tips on limiting your list of invitees, shortening the visits, and gaining some benefit from the intrusion:

- Discourage visitors with symptoms of a viral infection, such as a fever, runny nose, cough, rash, or diarrhea. Young children (unless they are your own) should avoid visiting or at least close contact with the new baby in the first month of life; they are often harboring a viral illness. Blame this rule on your doctor if people are offended.

- Let people know they should call before coming — this gives you some choice about what time is best for you and provides you with a bit of warning.
- When people ask what they can bring over, do not say "Nothing." Tell them dinner would be great!
- Ask all visitors to wash their hands as soon as they enter your house. You may want to place a container of antibacterial pump soap at your front door. Most viruses are transmitted through hand-to-hand contact.
- When your visitors arrive, put them to work! Once settled in, they can watch the baby while you have a quick shower, or they can clean your dirty dishes or get you something to drink. Real friends enjoy pitching in.
- Close family members who do not consider themselves to be visitors are often the worst offenders — set limits. You and your spouse may want some private time with your newborn away from parental advice. From the start, establish acceptable boundaries with your family members. Tell them what is really helpful and what is not so useful. They will usually get the message.

KEY POINT

Do not feel as if you have to entertain the entire world; if your visitors have children of their own, they will understand that the first few weeks are a period of adjustment and that eventually they will be able to meet your baby.

Playtime

During your baby's first month, most of his time and energy (and yours!) will be focused on feeding, sleeping, and growing. Even so, spending time interacting with him during awake and alert periods is important for his development and your developing relationship. A baby at this age might not seem to share your enthusiasm for the interaction, but he will still benefit from it.

Kinds of Play

Most of your play at this stage will consist of cuddling, rocking, singing, and talking to your newborn. He may spend periods of time gazing at an object or your face. Remember that his vision is not yet fully developed. In the first month, babies find it easiest to see large objects with strong contrast, such as black and white patterns or an adult's face close to theirs.

Your baby is also learning to understand the sounds he hears. Soft cooing, talking, and singing help him with this developmental task. As he grows, you will start to see him turning toward your voice. Soon, your baby will learn to distinguish your voice from a stranger's.

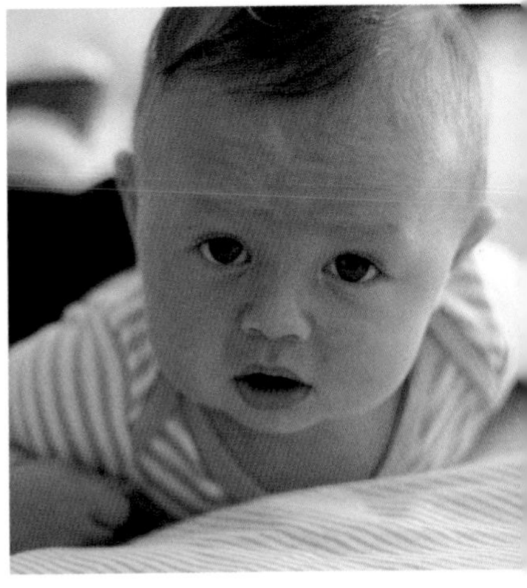

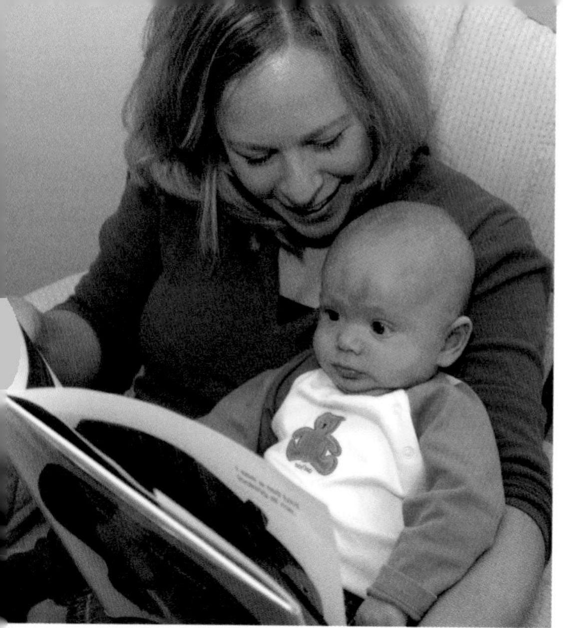

Reading to Your Baby

It is never too early to read to your baby. Reading plays an extremely important role in infant and child brain development. Even in the early stages when he doesn't understand the words, your baby will enjoy hearing your voice. Besides the tremendous stimulation it provides, reading encourages a close relationship between you and your baby. Don't be perturbed if he tries to eat the books or handles them roughly — that's why you start off with durable cloth or board books. Your baby may enjoy soft cloth books in black and white or in bright colors.

KEY POINT

Set aside a regular time each day to read to your baby.

Tummy Time

Because "Back to Sleep" programs recommend that babies be put to sleep on their backs to decrease the risk of sudden infant death syndrome (SIDS), babies may spend very little time on their tummies. As a result, they may lack the opportunity to develop the corresponding muscles.

To develop these muscles, "tummy time" is an important activity for babies. While he is awake, set your baby on his tummy for a few minutes at a time, several times per day, always under close supervision. Some babies will enjoy this time, while others will scream until they're picked up.

Don't force your baby into tummy time. Continue to try it regularly; eventually, your baby's head control and arm strength will allow him to feel more comfortable and happy in this position. Many parents find it helpful to put a mirror on the floor during tummy time. Lean over the mirror with your baby so that he can enjoy both of your reflections, which will gradually hold his attention for longer periods of time.

Bathing Playtime

Bath time and diaper changes (which are pretty often) are excellent opportunities to talk to, sing to, and tickle your baby. You want these activities to be fun in addition to fulfilling their function. They are also great times for other family members to get involved in playing and interacting with the baby, especially if they are unable to help with feeding.

Frequently Asked Questions

I have a newborn and two other young children. What is the best way to stop the spread of germs?

Frequent hand-washing with soap and water is still the most effective way to reduce the spread of germs. It is especially important if anyone has diarrhea or is vomiting, coughing, or sneezing. Remember to wash your hands and your children's hands after wiping noses and throwing away used tissues. Keep alcohol-based solutions and gels handy for those times when you aren't near a water source.

I love our new baby, but there seem to be too many moments when I'm tearful. What should I do?

It's easy to blame your sadness on simple fatigue. But that would be wrong. Many women experience significant depression following childbirth. Although postpartum depression is often transient and relatively mild, it can sometimes pose a serious risk to both mother and baby. It's important to discuss your feelings with your partner and your health-care provider. You should have no feelings of shame or guilt if you're suffering from postpartum depression — it is a common problem that can be treated.

I am a first-time parent and have lots to learn about babies. However, everyone seems determined to offer me advice, even when I don't want it. How do I handle well-meaning but unsolicited advice?

It sometimes seems that everyone who has ever had a baby thinks she's an expert on parenting. The best advice is usually asked for, not imposed upon you. Try to listen politely and evaluate each suggestion objectively. But in the end, this is your baby. Trust your own instincts about what works best for you and your child.

I've heard that formula with iron can cause constipation. If my baby is constipated, should I find a formula without iron?

Actually, all types of formula have some iron. Those advertised as "with iron" just have a higher concentration of it. The iron in "iron-fortified" formulas is important for the healthy development of young infants, and there is no good evidence to suggest that formula "with iron" will cause constipation.

I speak English and my husband speaks French. Is it a good idea to expose our baby to both languages from the beginning? I've heard different opinions.

You've heard different opinions because it is a matter of personal choice. Babies and young children are very quick to pick up languages, and even though they may mix them up a little initially, they will ultimately master both of them. A second language is often part of a family's history and culture, and this will be an important part of your baby's life in the future. Whether you start from birth or wait until your child is a few years old, use the second language as you do the first — interspersed in the regular activities of day-to-day life, including play and reading.

CHAPTER 5

Helping Your Baby Sleep

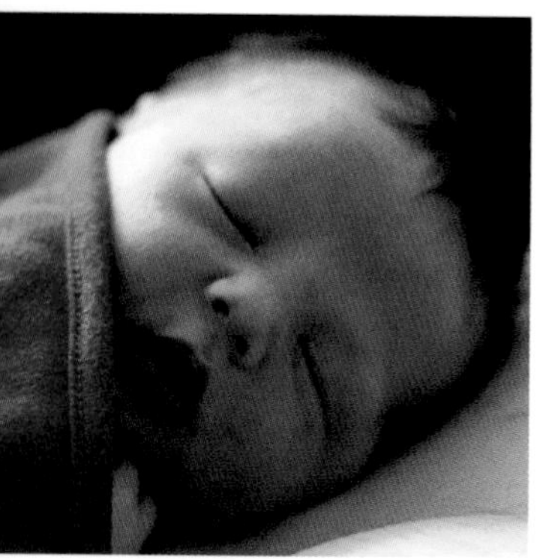

The birth of a new baby brings about many changes in a family's routine. One of the most distressing changes for parents is lack of sleep. Prior to the delivery of your baby, you probably received some "words of wisdom" on surviving with very little sleep, but only once you have your baby can you truly understand how precious a few hours of sleep can be.

There are many things you can do throughout your baby's first year of life to promote healthy sleep habits, starting as soon as your baby is born. The bad news is that your baby's sleep is very different from yours!

Functions of Sleep

Sleep is essential for the growth and development of your baby. Without sleep, our bodies cannot function properly. Sleep experts at the Hospital for Sick Children and elsewhere have identified several possible functions of sleep that promote good health:

- Restoration and regeneration of body systems
- Protection and recovery from infections
- Consolidation of memory
- Optimum daytime function of learning, memory, mood, attention, and concentration
- Growth and development of body and brain

Adapted with permission from Shelly K. Weiss, *Better Sleep for Your Baby & Child* (Toronto: Robert Rose, 2006).

Understanding Sleep

There are two main kinds of sleep: REM (rapid eye movement) and NREM (non–rapid eye movement) sleep.

REM Sleep

REM sleep is commonly referred to as "dreaming sleep." In REM sleep, your brain is in an active state, even though you are asleep. Under your eyelids, your eyes move rapidly. Your heart rate and breathing rate may also fluctuate. While your brain is very active, your body is very still, apart from small muscle twitches. In this state, it may be easier for someone to wake you up than if you were in NREM sleep.

In children, REM sleep is thought to help with the development of memory and contribute to learning.

NREM Sleep

NREM sleep is a deeper, more restorative kind of sleep. There are different degrees of NREM sleep, from light to deep. If you are in deep NREM sleep, you may feel confused or disoriented if someone wakes you up, and you may be difficult to rouse. This is the stage of sleep that allows a parent to carry a sleeping child from the car to the crib without the child waking. In this stage, your heart and breathing rate stay fairly consistent, and you do not dream as much as you do in REM sleep, because your brain is not as active.

In children, the purpose of this sleep is restoration of the body.

DID YOU KNOW?

"RESTLESS" SLEEP

Many parents are unaware of the different stages of sleep and often mistake normal sleep actions for discomfort or an unsettled baby. If your baby is in REM sleep (what we call active dreaming), she may smile, frown, suck, or twitch her limbs, and will be easily roused. She may appear to be restless, but she is actually just in a normal REM sleep phase. When your baby is in NREM sleep (restorative sleep), she will appear to be sleeping more deeply and will be more difficult to rouse.

Sleep Cycles

During an average night, your baby will go through several cycles of REM and NREM sleep. The duration of each cycle will change with growth and development. By the time an infant is about 6 months old, her sleep cycles will have changed to resemble those of an adult. Until this time, your baby may need more help from you to be able to sleep — you might comfort, hold, or rock her, for example. Once her sleep is more sophisticated, it is more reasonable to expect her to sleep on her own.

Partial Arousals

Newborns cycle through REM and NREM sleep about every 60 minutes, whereas adults do so every 90 to 110 minutes. At the end of each cycle, we all have a partial arousal. When this happens in infants, they will commonly fall back into a deeper sleep. Unfortunately, many parents mistake this arousal for an awakening and pick up their baby, causing a true awakening (full arousal) and disrupting the baby's sleep. If you do not teach your baby how to fall asleep on her own, these partial arousals may develop into full arousals throughout the night.

DID YOU KNOW?

KEEPING YOUR BABY AWAKE

Parents often believe that keeping a newborn baby awake during the day will help her sleep at night. This is not true. At this age, it will just make her fussier and unhappy, potentially worsening her sleep.

Circadian Rhythms

Circadian (24-hour) rhythms also play a part in regulating our sleeping and waking. Light and dark, eating patterns, physical activities, and hormones all affect our biological sleep rhythms, regulating when we feel sleepy and when we feel awake in a 24-hour period.

What Is Normal?

Most parents wonder how much sleep their baby really needs. Some parents feel their baby seems to sleep all the time, whereas others feel she is constantly awake and no one is getting any rest! So what is normal?

Sleep Patterns in the First Year

AGE	AVERAGE SLEEP TIME PER DAY	TYPICAL ROUTINE	COMMENTS
0 to 3 months	17 hours (15 to 20 hours)	• May wake to feed every 2 to 4 hours during the day and night. • Will be awake for 1 to 2 hours before falling asleep again.	• Sleep and wake cycles are often driven by hunger. • 50% of sleep typically occurs during the day.
3 to 6 months	15 hours (14 to 16 hours)	• May sleep through the night with 2 to 3 naps during the day. • Middle of the night feeding is usually eliminated during this phase.	• Setting up sleep routines becomes important so that your baby learns what to expect.
7 to 12 months	14 hours	• Should sleep through the night with 2 naps during the day lasting 30 minutes to 2 hours.	• Your baby should be able to soothe herself to sleep. • A short period of crying before falling asleep is normal, and not harmful. • Transitional objects (stuffed animal or "blankie") may help ease separation.

Developing Healthy Sleep Habits

Parents can help their babies become good sleepers by teaching them healthy sleep hygiene. Good sleep hygiene involves establishing a consistent sleep routine. This consistency is the key to preventing sleep problems.

Sleep Hygiene

The first few months require the development of a secure, nurturing environment for your new baby to sleep. Your baby's room should be consistently quiet, dark at night, comfortable, and cool, to promote sleep onset and maintenance. Your child should also have a consistent space — bassinet, crib, or bed — to sleep in during the night and at naptime, whether in your room, in a room with a sibling, or in her own room. If your baby wakes soon after falling asleep or in the middle of the night, she should be in the same environment she was in when she fell asleep. That way, she can replicate the skills used initially to fall asleep to go back to sleep.

Despite having a healthy sleep environment, your baby may wake up soon after falling asleep and during the night. This is not uncommon. All people, but especially babies, have the potential to wake up as they cycle into the lighter stages of sleep (partial arousal). Babies under 6 months of age have an even greater chance of waking because they spend more time in REM sleep than in NREM sleep. The key to preventing this normal sleep pattern from becoming a problem is to teach your child the skills needed to put herself to sleep and to remain asleep at night. This involves establishing a consistent bedtime and naptime routine.

Healthy Sleep Routines

Months 0 to 3

Hunger often drives the sleep-wake cycle of the newborn baby, but even at this age, consistency helps. Regular feeding schedules that complement sleeping schedules are useful. Feeding should be separate from sleeping, meaning that your baby should be awake when feeding (either by breast or bottle). Once she falls asleep, feeding should stop. If she is not finished a feeding, you may need to rouse her to complete the feeding. This will help her define distinct periods when she eats and when she sleeps, and she won't develop the habit of being able to fall asleep only when she is being fed.

Allowing your baby to fall asleep on her own at this age is just fine, but don't be surprised if she doesn't. You may need to hold her or rock her until she's sleepy. To

DID YOU KNOW?

GOOD SLEEPERS

Are some children inherently good sleepers, while others aren't? Yes, but this is no different from many things in life. Does this mean that some children are destined to sleep poorly? Not necessarily, especially if you give your child the right cues to learn to sleep. Sleep is somewhat innate, but it is also learned. Providing babies with a healthy sleep routine and teaching them how to put themselves to sleep without you will allow them to become "good sleepers."

KEY POINT

Letting your newborn cry herself to sleep is inappropriate. You should respond to the cries of a young infant during the first few months of life. For a newborn, crying is not manipulative behavior but rather her only way of communicating a need, such as feeding, diaper changes, or soothing.

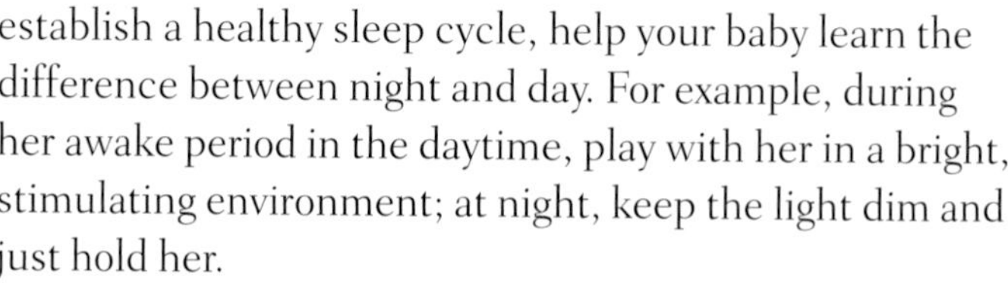

establish a healthy sleep cycle, help your baby learn the difference between night and day. For example, during her awake period in the daytime, play with her in a bright, stimulating environment; at night, keep the light dim and just hold her.

Months 3 to 6

As your baby grows and matures, you will notice that she is awake more often and is more aware of daytime and nighttime. Consistent routines are being learned. Continue to follow her cues when it comes to feeding. By 3 months of age, some babies will be sleeping through the night and will no longer need to be fed during the night. Sleeping patterns vary from baby to baby, and the evidence on sleeping through the night shows no difference between breast-fed and bottle-fed babies.

If possible, try to have your baby take naps in her crib. Stimulate and play with her during her daytime alert periods, but keep the lights low and your voice soft when she is awake at night. Her napping schedule and bedtime should start to take on some semblance of a routine. Try to determine when your little one is tired and put her into her crib while she is awake.

DID YOU KNOW?

SLEEPING THROUGH THE NIGHT

"Sleeping through the night" means sleeping for a period of 5 to 6 hours in a row, usually from midnight to 5 a.m. It doesn't mean sleeping from 7 p.m. to 7 a.m.! Also, infants have short sleep cycles (50 to 60 minutes), which means that during these 5 hours they may stir but are able to soothe themselves and put themselves back to sleep. If your baby doesn't sleep through the night at 3 months, don't worry. This is still well within the limits of normal. No intervention is necessary — just continue with your routines.

Months 7 to 12

By 6 months of age, your baby may sleep through the night (for a 5- to 6-hour stretch), but only if you have given her the tools to do so. Don't be disappointed if your 7-month-old still occasionally wakes up. Good sleeping takes practice.

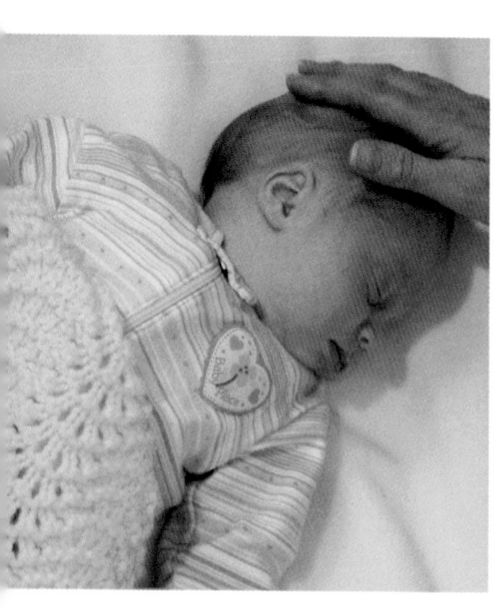

A 6-month-old baby will usually nap two to three times a day and then sleep for 10 to 12 hours at night, though not always continuously. Once your baby is 9 months old, she will likely have only two naps and may sleep through the night for 10 to 12 hours. If possible, your baby should nap at the same time every day and go to bed at the same time every night. In the morning, a well-rested baby will wake by herself.

By this age, children of a normal weight do not need to be fed during the night; they can safely go without feeds for 6 to 10 hours overnight. If you are feeding your baby during the night, you will need to wean her from these feeds slowly so that she isn't waking because she is hungry.

HOW TO: Establish a Healthy Sleep Routine

Although it is unreasonable to expect your 3-week-old baby to have a regular bedtime and naptime, there is evidence to show that instituting a consistent bedtime sleep routine from birth teaches your child the cues that sleep time is coming. Here are some tips to help you establish a healthy sleep routine from the start:

1. Before bedtime, create and maintain a quiet and relaxing atmosphere. Start by giving your baby a warm bath, feed her, change her into a fresh sleeper, read her a story, and sing your favorite songs.
2. After these comforting activities, place your awake or drowsy baby into her crib, giving her the opportunity to fall asleep on her own. Some children will be very good at this, while others will not, but practice makes perfect. Allowing your baby to try this over and over again will help her learn to fall asleep on her own, which will be particularly useful if she wakes up in the middle of the night.
3. For babies under 4 to 6 months, allow some fussing, but if your baby is crying consistently and hard, cuddle, hold, and soothe her before trying again to settle her in her crib.
4. After an hour or two, you may hear your baby move or fuss. Allow her the opportunity to put herself back to sleep before going in to check on her. This awakening is likely to be a partial arousal, an event that occurs every 60 minutes or so during sleep. Do not take it as a cue to awaken your child.
5. The same strategies for bedtime routines apply to naptime. Although a naptime routine does not generally include bathing, it should include placing your awake or drowsy baby in her crib to fall asleep. She will then learn that her crib is where she sleeps.
6. Some babies seem to need the warmth and comfort of their parents to sleep. Don't give up on consistent sleep routines and frequent attempts to place your awake baby in her crib — as she grows and develops, so will her sleep cycles and patterns. Sleep patterns become more organized in the second and third months of life.

Sleep-Stretching Techniques

These techniques can be used from birth to help your baby sleep for longer stretches at night. Their effectiveness will vary from baby to baby.

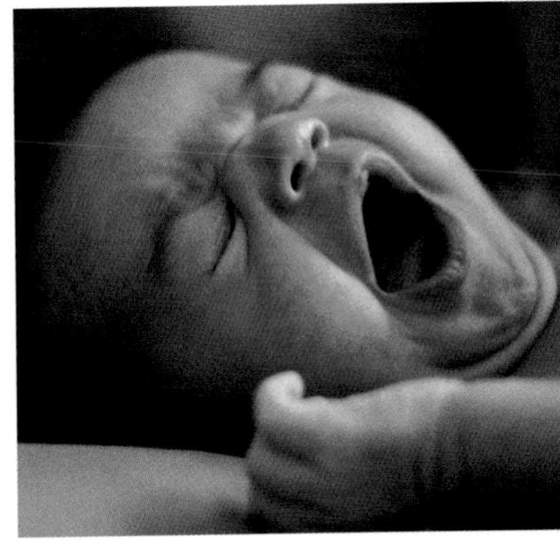

- **Focal feed:** Introduce a "focal feed," offered to the newborn each night between 10 p.m. and 12 a.m. Babies offered such a feed may sleep for longer periods during the night.
- **Nighttime cues:** Help your baby understand the difference between day and night. A dark, quiet

environment should cue a baby that it is night, while a bright, stimulating environment will let her know that it is daytime.

- **Non-feeding activities:** Respond to your baby's awakening during the night with a non-feeding activity, such as a diaper change or short walk. This helps to lengthen the time between feeds during the middle of the night. Studies have shown that babies who are treated in this way feed the same amount as other babies, with a longer early morning feed. This approach should only be tried once feeding is established (usually after 4 to 6 weeks).

> **DID YOU KNOW?**
>
> **CONSISTENT SLEEP TIMES**
>
> Before you establish a routine, you should be familiar with what time your baby usually goes to bed, wakes up, and naps. These times should remain consistent, even when your baby is up at night. For example, if she initially spends much of the night awake and crying, she should still be woken at her regular time and be kept awake until her regular naptime. This is sometimes very difficult — do the best you can. It is important to prevent your child from shifting her sleep schedule to sleep much longer during the day because she was awake all night.

Sleeping Safely

Creating a safe sleep environment for your baby involves choosing a sleeping style that reduces the risk of sudden infant death syndrome (SIDS) and nurtures your child in a family setting. You need to ask yourself where your baby will sleep — in your room, in her crib or your bed, or in her own room, in her crib or her bed? Your answer to these questions should be informed by an understanding of the benefits and risks of various sleeping arrangements, especially bed-sharing and co-sleeping.

Bed-Sharing and Co-sleeping

Many parents choose to share their bed with their infant; in fact, this is the most common sleeping arrangement among many cultures in many parts of the world. Even if you don't actually share a bed with your child, you may choose to sleep in close proximity, with your child beside your bed in her bassinet or crib so you can easily bring her into your bed to feed or to be soothed when she wakes in the night.

The American Academy of Pediatrics recommends a separate but close sleeping environment. Other medical experts feel that babies should be placed in their own rooms as soon as they come home from the hospital. This is a personal decision, and you may want to discuss it with your doctor.

Risks and Benefits

Bed-sharing has been shown to encourage and sustain breast-feeding, likely because it is less disturbing to a mother's sleep to nurse her baby in bed. However, studies have shown that bed-sharing, as practiced in North America and other developed countries, is more hazardous to your baby than sleeping in a separate crib or bassinet because there's a chance that adults will roll over and suffocate their babies.

One solution recommended by the American Academy of Pediatrics is to have an approved crib or bassinet in the parents' room, beside the parents' bed, for the first few months of life. This can facilitate breast-feeding and encourage close proximity to your baby while removing the potential risks of SIDS.

Other issues to consider include bed-sharing's effect on you and your partner, including the potential disruption of your sleep and your relationship.

Babies who co-sleep tend to breast-feed frequently during the night. When you decide to move your baby to her own crib, you may need to eliminate nighttime feeds and teach her new sleep associations. The transition from bed-sharing to sleeping in a crib is easiest on a relatively young baby (under 8 months).

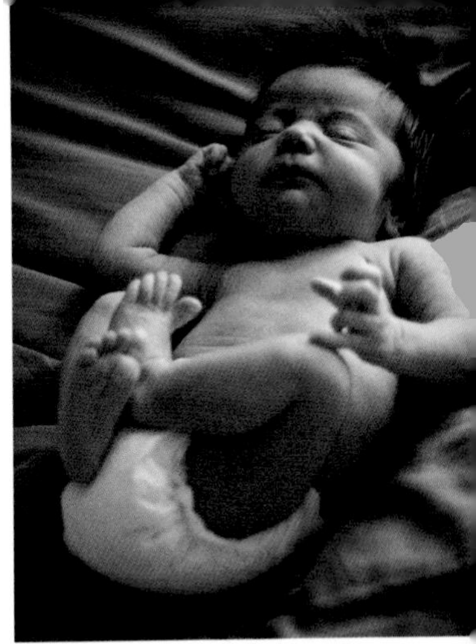

Reducing the Risk of SIDS

While we aren't sure about the cause of SIDS, there are a number of things that parents can try to do to minimize the risk.

- **Place your infant on her back.** Babies should be placed to sleep on their backs until they are old enough to roll over from the back to the tummy. Avoid products developed to maintain sleep position, such as foam positioning rolls or wedges.
- **Place infants on a firm sleeping surface without pillows, quilts, comforters, loose bedding, stuffed animals, or toys.** The American Academy of Pediatrics recommends against the use of bumper pads. If blankets are used, they should be thin and they should have holes.
- **Avoid bed-sharing.** The risks associated with bed-sharing are increased when a parent is a smoker, is under the influence of drugs or alcohol, or is extremely sleep-deprived (which, unfortunately, is the case for many new parents).

DID YOU KNOW?

SIDS

SIDS is defined as the sudden and unexpected death of an apparently healthy baby in the first year of life. As you may surmise from the "sudden and unexpected" part of the definition, this tragedy is not well understood. We don't really know the true cause, or causes, of SIDS. However, we do know that the risk reaches a peak at 2 to 3 months of age, and that 95% of cases occur in the first 6 months.

DID YOU KNOW?

BACK TO SLEEP

One big change in parental behavior over the last two decades has resulted from the "Back to Sleep" campaign, which recommends that babies sleep on their backs for the first 6 months to decrease the risk of SIDS. This does mean that a baby doesn't get much practice at developing her skills or strength while on her tummy; it may, therefore, take her a bit longer to get the strength to lift her head up, roll over, or crawl from the tummy-down position. To compensate, all babies should have some "tummy time" when awake.

- **Prevent your baby from overheating.** Your infant should be clothed for sleep as you are, with one or two layers of light clothing.
- **Don't smoke.** Smoke in the baby's environment is a risk factor for SIDS, and is harmful for other reasons (including asthma). Even if you do not smoke in the home, smoke particles cling to your clothing and hair.
- **Consider using a pacifier.** Studies have shown that pacifiers may decrease the risk of SIDS, though it is not clear how. However, some experts believe that pacifier use may interfere with breast-feeding; they therefore suggest that pacifiers be used when putting the baby to sleep only after breast-feeding is well established. The American Academy of Pediatrics suggests that a pacifier can be used when placing an infant to sleep for naps and at night, but should not be used if the infant does not want to take it and should not be replaced once the infant falls asleep.
- **Avoid home monitors.** Electronic monitors that measure your baby's movement, breathing, or heart rate, or sounds in your baby's room, do not help reduce the risk of SIDS and may create a false sense of security.
- **Continue breast-feeding.** Babies who are breast-fed have a lower risk of SIDS. Again, this relationship is not well understood.

Positional Plagiocephaly (Flat Head)

As a result of the successful "Back to Sleep" campaign, infants now have an increased incidence of positional plagiocephaly, or flat head — which sounds serious but generally isn't. If a baby spends most of her time on her back and prefers to look toward the left (for example, at a toy), then after a while the pressure of the firm mattress will cause the left side of her fairly soft, malleable skull to become somewhat flattened. The flattening often becomes visible around 3 to 4 months of age.

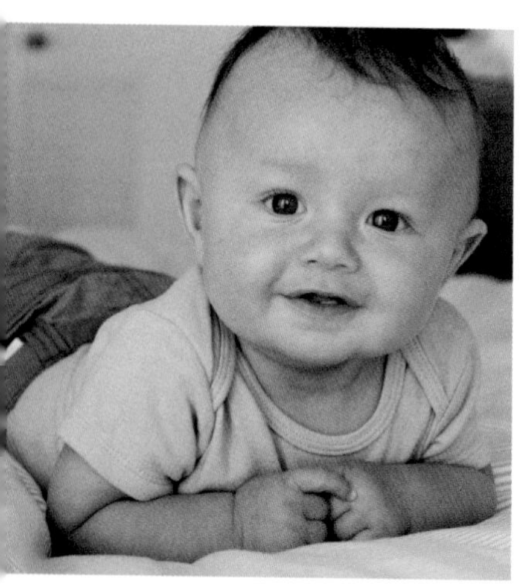

No baby's head is perfectly round, but if you notice a big difference between one side and the other, see your doctor. There is no real danger of abnormal brain growth or development, but in some very severe cases, your baby may need to wear a helmet that protects the skull and allows it to mold into a more rounded shape.

Other ways to prevent flat head include holding your baby in an upright position as much as possible and limiting her time on her back when she's awake. Try changing her sleeping position every day. This is easily achieved by placing your baby's head at the head of the crib one day and then toward the bottom of the crib the next day. Rotating the position of a favorite mobile is another easy strategy.

Treating Common Sleep Problems

There are two main types of sleep problems: those associated with difficulty getting to sleep or staying asleep (dyssomnias) and those that happen during sleep (parasomnias). Some examples of dyssomnias in young children are inappropriate sleep associations, frequent feeding through the night, and early awakenings. Parasomnias are defined as unusual behaviors while sleeping. In infants, these include rhythmic movements, such as head banging. As babies grow into toddlers, other common parasomnias include nightmares and night terrors.

Inappropriate Sleep Associations

Babies often develop sleep associations, or "props," to help them fall asleep. Parents are frequently the source of these associations. For example, if your baby always falls asleep while feeding, while listening to background music, or while her back is being rubbed, she might expect those conditions to be present each time she falls asleep. This may not be an issue at bedtime or naptime, but it becomes a *big* problem during the night, at the end of each sleep cycle, when she rouses and needs her prop to fall asleep again.

A baby with inappropriate sleep associations can awaken seven to eight times a night, leading to disrupted sleep for both the baby and her parents.

Improving Sleep Associations

The goal is to have your infant fall asleep on her own by teaching her appropriate sleep associations and removing inappropriate ones. Once she knows how to fall asleep on her own, her awakenings during the night will not become full awakenings. She will learn to soothe herself back to sleep.

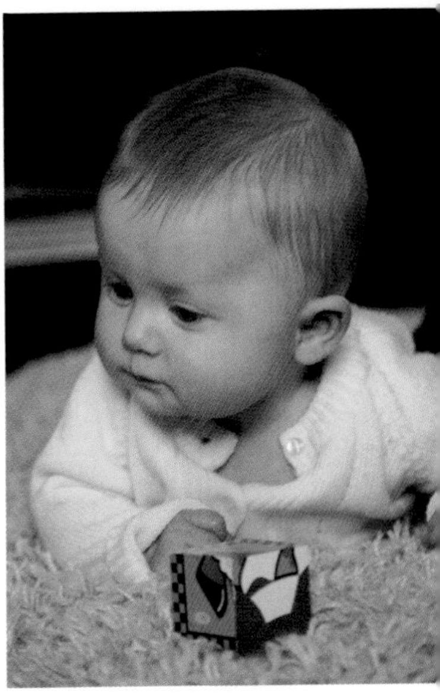

DID YOU KNOW?

TUMMY TIME

You can prevent flat head by encouraging your baby to spend time on her tummy while she is awake. Tummy time will also encourage good head control and upper body and shoulder strength. Many babies don't like tummy time at first because they are used to being on their back. Start by placing your baby on her tummy for 3 to 5 minutes at a time, several times a day, and gradually increase tummy time to at least 30 minutes a day. Try placing a brightly colored toy or a mirror in front of her to provide stimulation.

KEY POINT

Solving your baby's inappropriate sleep associations is not easy. Before embarking on a treatment plan, you and your partner must agree that a sleep problem exists and agree on the treatment approach. Making changes to your infant's behavior requires commitment, consistency, and fortitude. You and your partner, and all other caregivers, will need each other's support during the process.

Develop Appropriate Sleep Associations

1. Establish a bedtime routine. This should include gently talking to, holding, and cuddling your baby, but she should not be asleep when she is placed in her crib.
2. Put your baby into her crib while she is drowsy but awake.
3. Ensure that your baby falls asleep in a consistently comfortable, quiet, and dark environment. Put her to sleep in the same room, in the same crib, and in the same manner each night.

Remove Inappropriate Sleep Associations

1. If you have not already done so, wean your baby off her nighttime feeds (see page 122). She will learn to feed during the day and not awaken hungry at night.
2. If your baby has multiple sleep associations, remove them gradually, one at a time, day by day. For example, if your sleep routine is to walk your baby up and down the stairs, singing and rocking her to sleep, stop walking up and down the stairs for the first 2 to 3 nights. The next 2 to 3 nights, stop rocking her. Finally, for the last 2 to 3 nights, stop singing to her. It is perfectly appropriate to continue to rock and sing as part of your bedtime routine — just ensure that your baby is not falling asleep during these activities. Ultimately, you will put her into her bed while she is sleepy but awake.

Graduated Extinction

After inappropriate sleep associations are successfully removed, some babies learn to fall asleep on their own, but others need further guidance in the form of a behavioral therapy called graduated extinction. This method encourages self-soothing. Studies have shown graduated extinction to be effective in young infants, without any long-term negative side effects.

This approach is recommended for babies at least 4 to 6 months of age. The goal is to slowly increase the amount of time you leave your baby in her crib to fall asleep, to teach her how to soothe herself to sleep.

1. First, decide how long you will initially leave your baby in her crib — that is, how long you can stand to hear her cry. There is no magic number; some parents feel comfortable starting with 2 minutes, while others

are happy to go 5 minutes. The important thing is to be consistent.

For example, on Day 1, after you place your baby in her crib while she is sleepy but awake, she may be upset and start to cry. If your starting time is 2 minutes, leave the room (out of sight of your baby) and wait through 2 minutes of significant crying before checking on her. If she is still crying after 2 minutes (likely she will be), spend 1 to 2 minutes in her room, speaking to her in a calm, gentle voice, place her lying down if she is standing up in her crib, and say a gentle and firm good night.

2. Now leave her for 4 minutes. If she is still crying after 4 minutes (which will feel like a lifetime), enter her room again and check on her.
3. Next, increase your waiting time to 6 minutes, and then to 8 minutes, before checking on her. Repeat each 8-minute interval until she is asleep.
4. On Day 2, start by waiting for 4 minutes, then increase how long you wait by 2 minutes each time until a maximum time of 10 minutes is reached.

For the first several nights this process could go on for up to 2 hours!

Repeat the process for up to 7 days. By then, even the most strong-willed baby will get the message and fall asleep on her own.

KEY POINT

When you check on your baby, do not inadvertently introduce new sleep associations: do not feed, hold, or rock her. The interaction should be short and reassuring. This routine should be repeated for all naps and bedtimes. Be consistent. All caregivers should use the same approach, both during the day and at night.

Frequent Nighttime Feeding

Babies who need to feed frequently through the night often have sleep-onset associations; that is, they associate falling asleep with feeding and need to feed to get back to sleep. This issue can affect babies who are bottle-fed or breast-fed. They often fall asleep easily with feeds, but wake up during the night appearing hungry and crying until they are fed. They may have excessively wet diapers during the night, leading to more wakenings and, subsequently, more feedings. Babies with this dyssomnia may feed three to nine times during the night.

Many parents consider this sleep issue to be problematic after 6 months of age. The first step in solving it is to reduce the number of times the baby is feeding during the night. Once the baby has learned to satisfy her nutritional needs during the day, she can learn to fall asleep without feeding.

HOW TO: Wean Your Baby from Nighttime Feedings

This approach can be introduced at 6 months of age. Like any other behavioral treatment, make sure your partner knows and agrees with the plan; you will need to be consistent, and you will need to support each other for this to work. If your baby has difficulty with weight gain or growth, consult your doctor for advice before you change her feeding schedule.

1. Establish a bedtime routine.
2. Determine how much feeding your baby does during the night. For 2 to 3 nights, keep a diary of each night awakening and feeding. If you are breast-feeding, record how many minutes your baby feeds on each breast for each feed.
3. Determine the average or typical amount of food your baby takes in overnight. For breast-feeding, calculate the average amount of time your baby feeds per feed, in minutes.
4. Decrease the breast or bottle feeds gradually. If you are breast-feeding, decrease the length of time per feed by 1 minute each night. For example, if you were breast-feeding on average for 8 minutes per feed, then decrease this to 7 minutes per feed the first night, 6 minutes per feed the second night, and so on until you are not feeding at night. If you are bottle feeding, decrease the amount by ½ ounce (15 mL) each feed per night. Depending on the length of time or amount of feeds your baby is taking, this step should take 7 to 14 days to complete.
5. It may be slightly more difficult for your baby to fall asleep during this process. Help her fall asleep by holding, rocking, or singing to her.
6. Be strong. This process may be exhausting in the short term, but remember, you are providing the guidance your baby needs to have a more restful sleep and consume her required calories during the day.
7. Let your baby drink for longer periods of time or consume a larger amount of formula during the day and at bedtime. This ensures that she will receive the right amount of food, just at a better time.

Early Awakening

Some babies develop very early awakening times, all of a sudden waking up at 5 a.m. on a daily basis, bright-eyed and ready to play. This may be your baby's normal sleep-wake pattern, and all efforts to ward off early morning awakenings may be futile. Your baby may have altered her biological clock and circadian rhythms. Unfortunately, you may need to learn to cope with this sleep pattern. But sleep patterns change frequently in the first year of life, and this pattern might too.

Coping with Early Awakening

If early awakening is a problem for your family, you will likely have to go back to the basics on sleep patterns and sleeping environment.

- Ensure that your baby's room is dark and quiet by blocking out the sun and outside noise.
- Record your child's sleep patterns for a 2- to 3-day period. Think about how her sleep patterns might have changed recently. For example, is she going to sleep earlier or taking a late-afternoon nap? She may be going to bed too early, or even too late. This may be her way of telling you that she doesn't need a late-afternoon nap (if she is still napping twice in the afternoon) or that she doesn't need a morning nap.
- Sometimes, her schedule hasn't changed; she is just waking up early and then needing an earlier morning nap. For example, if your baby is waking up at 5 a.m., she may also be napping from 8 to 9 a.m. In this situation, try to keep her awake until her regular morning nap at 10 a.m. If her naps seem appropriate, her bedtime may be too early; try moving it 10 minutes later each night for several nights until she begins to awaken later in the morning.
- If all else fails, keep a safe baby toy or book in her crib and encourage her to play alone for a while, to give you an extra few minutes in the morning.

DID YOU KNOW?

RHYTHMIC MOVEMENTS

When babies fall asleep, they sometimes develop a soothing repetitive motion, such as rocking their bodies or banging their heads. These movements can be seen as the baby is first falling asleep at night and during the normal frequent arousals overnight. They usually last less than 10 minutes and cause no harm to the baby. Although these movements may look strange or disturbing to parents, they are soothing and pleasurable to babies. They do not interfere with sleep or development, and they usually resolve during the toddler years.

Frequently Asked Questions

I am worried that my baby may stop breathing overnight. Several friends have suggested that I buy a baby monitor to prevent SIDS.

SIDS is a very rare condition that is not fully understood. What we do know is that we can significantly reduce the risk of SIDS by placing babies to sleep on their backs on a firm mattress without pillows or heavy blankets, and by avoiding exposing them to smoke and overheating. Baby monitors that measure movement, sound, breathing, or heart rate have not been shown to reduce the risk of SIDS. They are not recommended because they increase anxiety in families and usually result in less sleep for both babies and parents due to constant false alarms!

I place my baby to sleep on her back, but over the last week I have noticed that she rolls onto her tummy. Should I be rolling her over onto her back again?

Placing a baby to sleep on her back has been shown to decrease the risk of sudden infant death syndrome (SIDS). However, once a baby has started to roll over from back to front, there is no advantage to turning her back over. The risk of SIDS is reduced significantly by 6 months of age, likely related in part to a baby's ability to roll herself over and lift her head effectively.

My baby is almost 4 months old and is still waking up at 4 a.m. to feed. What can I do to get her to sleep through the night?

Don't be discouraged — many parents with a 4-month-old would be happy if they only had to get up once a night to feed her. "Sleeping through the night" at 4 months of age is considered to be a 5- to 6-hour stretch at one time. Try a focal feed (see page 115) and see if it helps. Also ensure that you are giving your baby a chance to learn how to soothe herself to sleep by putting her to bed while she is drowsy but awake.

My 9-month-old is still waking every 3 hours to feed at night. I think it is just a habit, but my husband feels he needs to be fed at night until he is a year old.

Your baby does not physiologically need to be fed at night if he is of a normal weight for his age. You can confirm this with your health-care provider. The majority of babies (unless they have medical problems) do not need to feed at night after 5 to 6 months of age. In fact, it is best for your son's growth and development if he sleeps through the night so he can benefit from the restorative functions of sleep. As you gradually start to wean him off nighttime feedings, he will start to eat more during the day.

My 7-month-old daughter has difficulty falling asleep at night. My friend recently told me to play soft classical music to help her. Is this something tried and true?

Definitely not! While having your baby listen to music during the day may be beneficial, listening while she falls asleep only creates an inappropriate sleep association that you will need to correct in the future. Your daughter's sleeping environment and sleep routines may give you clues as to why she is having trouble falling asleep.

Every time we go away on vacation, I regret it. My 11-month-old son seems to sleep okay while we are away, but once we return home, he reverts to his old routine, needing me to cuddle him back to sleep four or five times per night. Is this normal?

This is very normal. Many parents end up reteaching their children how to fall asleep by themselves once they return from vacation. When families go on vacation, everyone's sleep environment changes, with new bedrooms and beds. Your baby may adjust to sleeping in the same room as you when he was previously used to being in his own room, or, if you are in a hotel, you may not be able to allow him to cry at night. These changes result in poor sleep behaviors once you return from vacation. Reinstitute his sleep routine. With consistency, your son will quickly revert back to his good sleep pattern.

CHAPTER 6

Your Baby's Months 2 to 6

By your baby's second and third months, you are likely becoming more comfortable with your role as a parent and increasingly savvy at interpreting your baby's cues. Some infants of this age will naturally settle into a routine, around which you can begin to plan your day, even doing some things for yourself! By now, you have probably been to visit your baby's doctor a couple of times to measure your baby's growth, assess his development and start vaccinating him against infectious diseases. And as the exhaustion from the first month begins to wane, you may start to find that playing with your baby can be fun as his unique personality begins to emerge.

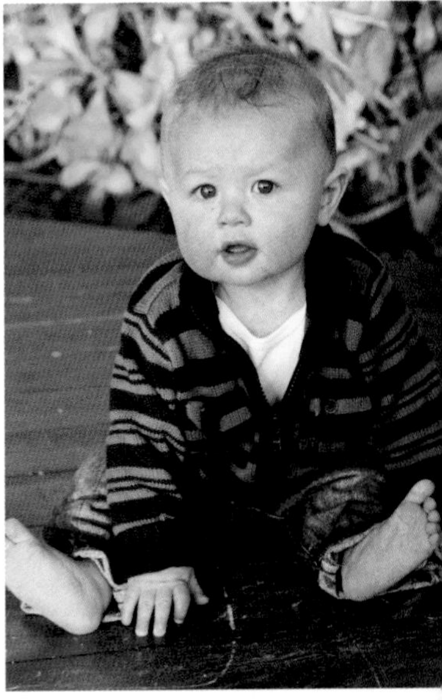

Establishing a Routine

The relative importance of routines largely depends on personality. Some parents thrive on structure and are anxious for their baby to have a schedule, while others are happy to live with unpredictable days for a while longer. If you crave structure but your baby's days remain inconsistent, you can try to implement a consistent routine. If you enjoy a carefree lifestyle, appreciate it for as long as you like, but keep in mind that the older your baby is when you establish a routine, the more difficult it will be to implement.

When establishing a routine, it is best to base it on your baby's cues and natural rhythms. These will differ in each infant; there is no right or wrong schedule. Ultimately, though, his needs — adequate nutrition, rest, and alert time — must come first. Responding to your baby's needs will establish security and trust.

KEY POINT

Everyone adjusts to life with a young infant at a different pace. Speak to your doctor or your child's pediatrician if you feel you are struggling to cope — they can help ensure you get the support you need.

Cyclical Patterns

A baby's routine involves feeding, sleeping, and times when he is awake and alert. These activities will often fall into a cyclical pattern. The length of the cycle will initially be dictated by the interval between feedings, usually every 2 to 3 hours at first, and then gradually longer intervals. Your baby's periods of being awake and alert will gradually lengthen and, as he grows, will evolve into times when you can really enjoy interacting. Use the time when your baby is sleeping to do things for yourself — such as taking a shower!

KEY POINT

Take care to avoid allowing your baby to fall asleep while feeding. It is natural for newborns to become sleepy during feeds, but if this becomes habit, your baby will associate the bottle or breast with falling asleep, which might contribute to sleep problems later on.

Bedtime Routine

Between 2 and 3 months, many babies begin to sleep for longer stretches at night. You can encourage this desirable habit by initiating a bedtime routine. A consistent bath time and singing a lullaby at bedtime, for example, will signal to your baby that it's time to say good night. Of course, at this age it is not unusual for babies to still require one or two nighttime feeds, but learning to differentiate night from day is a big step toward a good night's sleep for all.

Medical Checkups

Your baby will continue to have regular checkups — usually at 2, 4, and 6 months of age. Some doctors schedule routine visits at 3 months as well. Although it may seem like you are at the doctor's office all the time, frequent checkups are necessary during these early months because your baby is growing and changing so quickly.

While each health-care provider has a different style, the issues covered during these checkups are pretty much the same. You will be asked how your baby is feeding, sleeping, voiding, and stooling, as well as questions related to his development. Pediatricians learn very early on that a parent's instincts are usually extremely accurate, even with a first child. So share your observations and any concerns you have. The physician will see your baby for only a brief time and may not be able to observe that he is not focusing on an object or responding appropriately to noises, even if this is the case. Your answers alone will give your doctor a good idea of how your baby is progressing.

Your health-care provider will likely ask how the family is coping with your new bundle of joy — and the cause of your sleep deprivation. Be honest about what you are feeling and how you are coping. Your doctor may be able to give you advice or practical tips, or, if necessary, refer you to someone who can help if you aren't coping as well as you'd like.

If your baby is due for an immunization, it is usually given at the end of the appointment.

DID YOU KNOW?

ANTICIPATORY GUIDANCE

In addition to answering your questions, your physician will likely also offer anticipatory guidance about what to expect in the coming months, sometimes including advice about safety or public health concerns, such as car seat and bathtub safety, as well as immunizations.

Examining Your Baby

Your baby will have a full examination at each visit. Depending on his age and temperament, he may not mind being placed on the examining table, but your doctor can do much of the exam with your baby in your lap. Try to dress your baby in something that is easy to slip on and off — you don't want to be concentrating on closing all the snaps when you have important questions to ask.

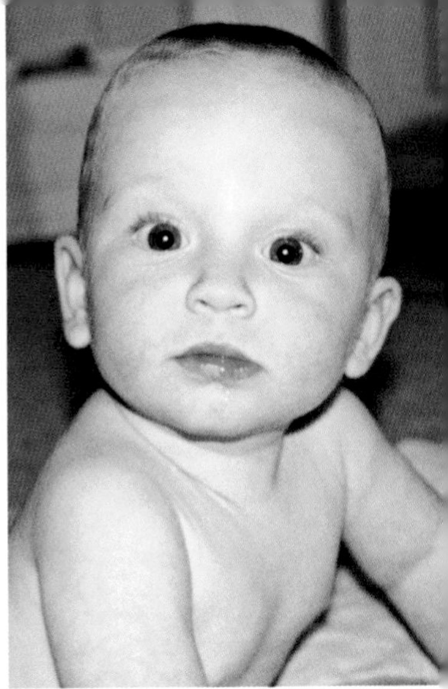

Measuring Your Baby Again

Your baby's weight will be taken on an infant scale, and his length and head circumference measured. All three measurements will be plotted on a growth chart, which is kept in your infant's medical record. While some babies are naturally big and others small, this chart will allow your doctor to ensure that your baby is growing at an appropriate rate.

Booking Appointments

To ensure that you keep up-to-date, ask your health-care provider at the end of each visit when she would like to see your baby next, and make an appointment on your way out. Some offices have specific times set aside in which to see "well babies." Take advantage of this to minimize the likelihood of exposing your young baby to illnesses while you're in the waiting room. If possible, schedule the visit for early in the day, when waiting time is usually shorter. Make sure you know whom to call after hours and what to do if you have questions before your next scheduled appointment.

> **KEY POINT**
>
> **Bring a written list of questions with you to make the most of your time with the doctor.**

Still Growing and Developing

Your baby's growth will be measured and plotted on a growth curve at least three times during the first 6 months (2, 4, and 6 months are the most common times), and more frequently if any concerns have been raised.

Growth Curves: 2 to 6 Months

Weight

By 2 months of age, an average North American baby weighs between 9 and 14 pounds (4 and 6.4 kg) and measures 21 to 25 inches (53 to 63 cm). Gains in weight continue at an average of ⅔ to 1 ounce (20 to 30 g) per day, slowing slightly toward the end of the first 6 months.

KEY POINT

Remember that growth can and does occur in spurts, so weight gain measured on a day-to-day basis is not as helpful as the progression over weeks and months. Your doctor will watch to ensure that your baby is growing at the expected rate based on his growth curve.

By 6 months, your baby has likely doubled in weight since he was born!

Height

Gains in height also continue, though at a slightly slower rate. By 6 months, an average baby measures between 24.5 and 28.5 inches (63 and 72 cm).

Head Circumference

Rapid brain growth continues, as demonstrated by your baby's head growth, which increases on average 0.5 inch (1 cm) every 2 weeks for the first 3 months and 0.5 inch (1 cm) every month between 3 and 6 months.

Development Milestones: 2 to 3 Months

Head Control

As the second and third months progress, your baby gradually becomes stronger. You will notice that he is gaining some control of his head. When you hold him against your shoulder or place him on his tummy, he will start to raise his head on his own and move it from side to side. However, if you pull him up to a sitting position, his back will remain rounded and his head will lag behind — he is not yet strong enough to support it completely.

DID YOU KNOW?

HOLDING OBJECTS

Although your baby's hands are held open more frequently now, he is not yet ready to hold objects. A block or rattle placed in his hand will fall right out again. He is also not quite ready to reach out for objects — don't worry, these skills will come soon.

Alertness

Throughout these months, your baby will become more alert. He will turn his head to follow your face or an interesting object, will quiet briefly when you speak softly to him, and will turn to look toward a noise. When picked up or stimulated, he will respond with smiles and excited movements.

Development Milestones: 4 to 6 Months

This is a period of rapid motor development. Your baby may now start to become more mobile! Most babies of this age are able to roll over independently; near the end of this period, a few may even start to crawl.

Head Control

By 4 months, head control has usually become established. When pulled up to a sitting position from lying on his back, your baby will support his own head. An infant is now able to lift his shoulders and head when lying on his tummy. As he gets stronger, he will be able to support his weight on his outstretched arms and, eventually, on his hands and knees. By 5 months, many infants are able to sit briefly if supported, and by 6 to 7 months, most babies are able to sit up alone for short periods.

Reaching and Holding

By 4 months of age, babies start to reach for and hold interesting objects. You can help your baby's development in this area by placing him on his back with interesting toys for him to reach toward. You can also try using an infant chair or "exersaucer" with a variety of different-shaped and colored objects for him to reach for, touch, and manipulate.

As your baby gains practice and dexterity, typically by 6 months, he will be able to transfer objects from one hand to the other. All objects seem to find their way eventually into his mouth, so beware of small ones he could choke on or swallow, or anything that has small appendages that are not tightly fastened, such as buttons or the eyes on teddy bears.

Conversation

Just as his motor skills are taking off, you will also notice a change in your baby's sounds. By 4 months, your baby will probably have a "conversation" with you; that is, if you imitate his sounds, he will answer back with another sound. He is learning that sounds have meaning!

By 6 months, these sounds will change from cooing vowel-based sounds to babbling sounds that include vowels and consonants, such as "da-da-da-da" or "ba-ba-ba-ba." Your delighted response and imitation of these sounds will encourage his language development.

Stranger Anxiety

Infants of this age begin to discriminate between parents and strangers and may seem wary of adults they don't know well. This is known as stranger anxiety. Don't worry, it's normal — though Grandpa may get upset when your baby cries at the sight of him.

DID YOU KNOW?

OBJECT PERMANENCE

At this age, your baby will enjoy looking at and manipulating toys — and putting them in his mouth — but he probably has not yet developed "object permanence," the recognition that an object no longer directly in view still exists. So, if he drops a toy, he won't yet look to see where it went.

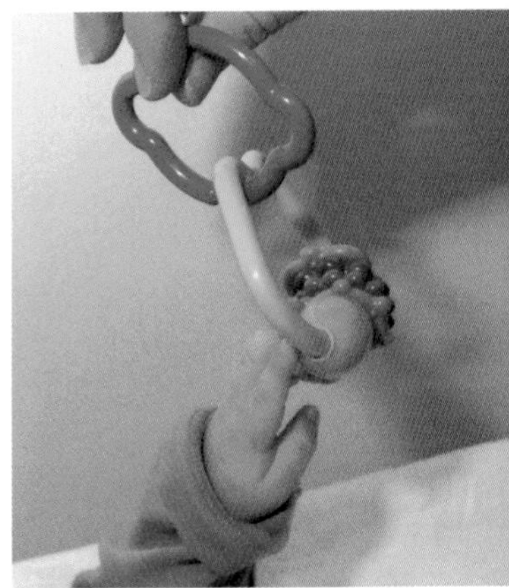

KEY POINT

At around 4 months of age, babies start to put everything in their mouths. Ensure that all small objects are out of reach or well secured to prevent choking.

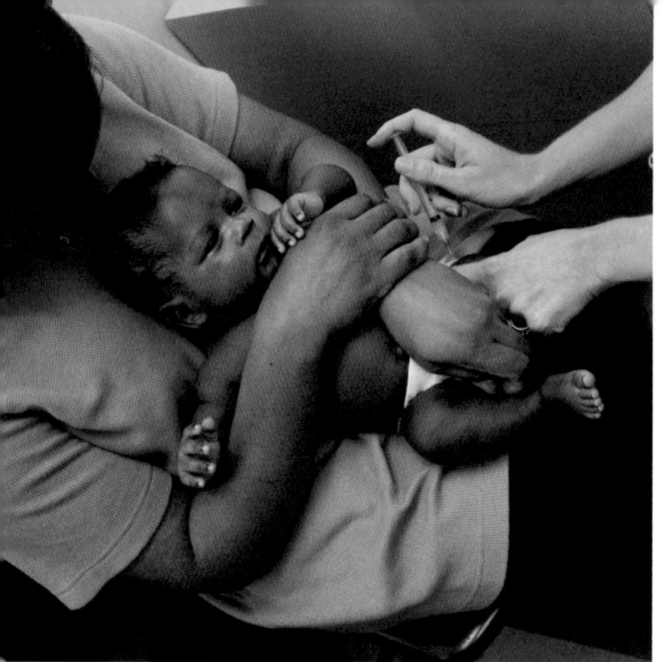

All About Vaccinations

An important part of well-baby visits in the first year is immunizations. With the advent of vaccines over the past 60 years, infectious diseases that previously caused sickness and death in many children are now rarely seen. Unfortunately, these illnesses have not been eradicated entirely, so unprotected children and adults remain vulnerable to them. Ensuring that your baby receives his vaccinations is one of the best preventive health measures you can provide.

Vaccine Safety

Many parents are concerned about the safety of the vaccines themselves. In fact, based on scientific evidence and the experience accumulated through millions of children immunized, immunizing your child is actually very safe. Your baby may experience some redness or soreness at the site where the needle was given, and, depending on the vaccine, a fever or rash is possible, but more serious side effects are exceedingly rare. Once the immediate discomfort of the needle has passed, most babies are not bothered at all. You may give your baby a pain medication, such as acetaminophen, to minimize side effects. If you are breast-feeding your baby, he may be comforted by nursing soon afterwards.

DID YOU KNOW?

SICK BABY

If your child has a cold, it is usually okay to go ahead with the immunization, though vaccines are typically deferred if a child has a fever or is very unwell.

Administration

Immunizations are usually reserved for the end of your doctor's visit, and may be given by either the physician or the nurse. Until babies are walking, the shots are typically administered in the thigh muscle. Following his physical exam, get your baby partially dressed, with his leg exposed, and hold him in a sitting position on your lap. Your doctor or nurse will hold his leg, clean the site with an alcohol swab, quickly administer the injection, and cover it with a Band-Aid.

Many immunization schedules require that two or more shots be given at the same visit. They are administered at different sites (one in each leg, for example), and this is a perfectly safe practice.

Immunization Cards

The specific immunization schedule varies between countries and provinces or states, but in most developed nations, the same coverage and protection is generally achieved. Be sure to discuss your baby's vaccination program with your health-care provider soon after your baby is born. Your physician or nurse will give you an immunization card that records your baby's vaccinations. Bring it with you to subsequent doctor's visits so you can keep track of your baby's shots. In the future, you will likely need to show it to child-care facilities such as daycares, schools, and camps. It is also important to take it with you if you are seeking health care from anyone other than your regular doctor (for example, the emergency room of your local hospital).

DID YOU KNOW?

ADDITIONAL VACCINATIONS

If you plan to travel with your baby (particularly to developing countries), or if any household member has a particular disease, such as hepatitis B, other vaccinations may be required in addition to the routine series.

DTaP Vaccine

DTaP is the abbreviation for a vaccine that immunizes your baby against diphtheria, tetanus, and acellular pertussis.

- **Diphtheria** is caused by bacteria, resulting primarily in difficulty breathing and heart and nerve problems. Babies who get diphtheria have a significant chance of dying from it.
- **Tetanus** (lockjaw) occurs when the tetanus bacterium, found in soil, gets into an open cut in the skin. Painful muscular spasms occur, the muscles that affect breathing may be affected, and long-term neurological problems may result. Thankfully, immunization and proper hygiene practices have made tetanus very uncommon in developed nations.
- **Pertussis** (whooping cough) is caused by bacteria that enter the lungs and cause a severe cough. Pertussis remains relatively common. Many adults lose their immunity to it over time and develop pertussis in the subtle form of a persistent cough; they can then pass the germ on to their baby. Young babies with pertussis may become critically ill and can even die if their cough becomes so severe that they have trouble breathing. In older children, the cough can last up to 3 months.

DID YOU KNOW?

5-IN-1 VACCINE

In Canadian jurisdictions, a "5-in-1" vaccine is available to protect your baby from five diseases: diphtheria, tetanus, pertussis, polio, and Hib. It is given at approximately 2, 4, and 6 months of age, and again at 18 months. In the United States, DTaP, Hib, and IPV are given at similar intervals, but in separate injections.

Hib Vaccine

This vaccine immunizes against *Haemophilus influenzae* type B, a bacterium associated with many childhood

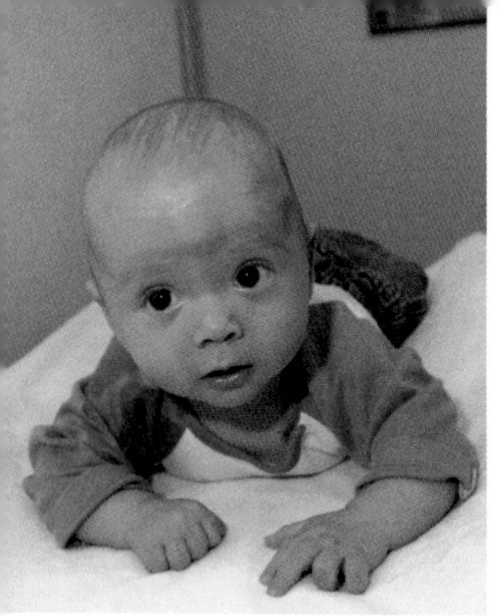

infections. Hib was previously one of the most common causes of meningitis, a potentially devastating infection of the brain and spinal cord. Since the vaccine was developed in the early 1990s, Hib is very rarely seen as a cause of such serious infections.

IPV Vaccine

The inactivated polio virus (IPV) vaccine will protect your baby from the polio virus. Many people infected with polio have very few symptoms, while others experience fever, headache, vomiting, muscle pain, and weakness. Some children even develop permanent paralysis. Prior to the widespread use of the vaccine, entire hospital wards were filled with children afflicted with polio who needed an "iron lung" respirator in order to breathe.

Chicken Pox (Varicella) Vaccine

Chicken pox is a common illness caused by the varicella-zoster virus. Chicken pox often causes a fever and an itchy rash. It can also have complications such as scarring, skin and blood infections, pneumonia, and inflammation of the brain. Chicken pox can be severe and even life-threatening in young babies, adults, and those with immune problems. It is recommended that children receive their first vaccine after the first year of life, followed by a booster dose at 4 to 6 years of age. This latter dose can be given as one needle in combination with the measles, mumps, and rubella (MMR) vaccine.

Hepatitis A Vaccine

This virus causes an acute, self-limited illness usually associated with fever, nausea, fatigue, jaundice, and loss of appetite. Infection is spread from person to person through ingestion of anything contaminated with infected feces, including inadequately treated drinking water. In the United States, the hepatitis A vaccine is recommended for all children at 1 year of age (two doses, 6 to 18 months apart).

Hepatitis B Vaccine

Hepatitis B is a virus that can affect the liver. If a mother carries the virus, it can be transmitted to her baby at birth. Other routes of transmission are from infected blood

DID YOU KNOW?

INFLUENZA VACCINE

Influenza is the virus that causes "the flu," common in the late fall and winter months. The flu can cause serious lung disease, particularly in those at high risk — young children, the elderly, and people with chronic medical conditions such as asthma or diabetes. The flu vaccine is given annually in the fall to those over 6 months of age, but is not mandatory. It works to lessen the frequency and severity of the infection. Speak to your health-care provider about a flu shot for your baby.

products, sexual contact with an infected individual, and injection drug use. The hepatitis B vaccine is given in a series of three shots, usually over a 6-month period. Depending on where you live, the vaccine is given beginning either at birth or in early adolescence.

Meningococcal C Conjugate Vaccine

Meningitis gets a lot of press when outbreaks occur in college residences, but babies less than a year old may also be at risk. This vaccine protects against one strain (type C) of meningococcus, a bacterium that causes meningitis and life-threatening blood infections. In the United States, this vaccine is not recommended in infancy, but is given at 11 to 12 years of age. The Public Health Agency of Canada recommends that children receive one dose at 12 months of age, and a dose of another meningococcal vaccine (Men-C-ACYW-135) that covers a wider number of strains in early adolescence.

MMR Vaccine

MMR stands for measles, mumps, and rubella. These three diseases, all caused by viruses, are covered by one vaccine. Two doses are needed — the first at 12 months and the second at least 1 month later, but usually at the age of 4 to 6 years.

- **Measles** (red measles) causes fever, runny nose, cough, red eyes, and a rash. In some children with measles, the virus affects the brain, with serious consequences.
- **Mumps** results in fever, headache, and painful swelling of the mouth's salivary glands. It can also cause meningitis and deafness.
- **Rubella** (German measles) causes fever, rash, and swollen glands. Pregnant women who contract rubella have a high chance of passing it on to their babies, which can be very serious. Depending on the stage of pregnancy when the fetus is infected with rubella, it can result in blindness, deafness, heart problems, or death. If you are thinking about getting pregnant and did not have the vaccine or the disease when you were a child, speak to your health-care provider about getting it now. This immunization cannot be given once you are pregnant.

KEY POINT

At one time, there was great concern that the MMR vaccine was associated with and, in fact, caused autism. However, large studies have proved that such concern is completely unfounded: the MMR vaccine does not cause autism.

Pneumococcal Conjugate Vaccine

This vaccine will protect your baby from *Streptococcus pneumoniae*, a common bacterium that causes meningitis, blood infections, pneumonia, and ear infections. These illnesses affect an enormous number of children, and, despite antibiotics, infections such as meningitis can still cause permanent brain damage or death. This vaccine is given as a series of three or four injections over the first 12 to 15 months, depending on the jurisdiction.

Rotavirus Vaccine

Rotavirus is the most common cause of gastroenteritis, which can cause fever, vomiting, and diarrhea. The vaccine is given as two to three doses (depending on the brand used) at 2, 4, and 6 (if a third dose is given) months. Rotavirus vaccine is given as a liquid by mouth.

Recommended Immunization Schedule for Infants

Age at vaccination	DTaP	IPV	Hib	MMR	Var	Hep B	Hep A	Pneu-C	Men-C	Flu	Rota
Birth						● 3 doses during infancy or in schools ✻ 3 doses: birth, 1–2 months, 6–18 months or in schools					
2 months	● ✻	● ✻	● ✻					● ✻	●		✻
4 months	● ✻	● ✻	● ✻					● ✻	●		✻
6 months	● ✻	● ✻	● ✻					●	●	● ✻ 6–59 months, given yearly	
12 months	● 18 months ✻ 6–18 months	● 18 months ✻ 12–18 months	● 18 months ✻ 12–15 months	● ✻ 12–18 months	● ✻ 12–18 months		✻ 12–23 months: 2 doses, 6 months apart	● ✻ 12–15 months			

DTaP: Diphtheria, tetanus, acellular pertussis

IPV: Inactivated polio virus vaccine

Hib: *Haemophilus influenzae* type B conjugate vaccine

MMR: Measles, mumps, and rubella vaccine

Var: Varicella-zoster virus (chicken pox) vaccine

Hep B: Hepatitis B vaccine

Hep A: Hepatitis A vaccine

Pneu-C: Pneumococcal conjugate vaccine

Men-C: Meningococcal C conjugate vaccine

Flu: Influenza vaccine

Rota: Rotavirus vaccine

● Recommended in the United States, as adapted from the Department of Health and Human Services, Centers for Disease Control and Prevention.

✻ Recommended in Canada, as adapted from the National Advisory Committee on Immunization, Public Health Agency of Canada.

Temperament

At 4 months of age, individual personality and temperament start to rapidly emerge. Babies at this stage become very interested in the world around them, and particularly in the people who hold and feed and smile at them. Parents, with their improving skills and growing confidence, find this period easier, and even fun.

KEY POINT

"Temperament" refers to how individuals naturally respond to people and situations. An individual's temperament is largely determined very early in life; temperament may even be innate. How parents react to their baby's temperament is critical, not just for this period but for a lifetime of parenting.

Easy and Difficult Children

The elements of temperament often occur in recognizable patterns. Some infants can be labeled "easy children." Their temperament allows them to adapt easily to most situations; they quickly fall into recognizable routines that simplify their care; and they usually seem happy. Such infants are a joy to parent.

Not every father and mother is so lucky. At the other end of the spectrum lies the "difficult child." These babies are intense; they dislike change; they have trouble establishing routines; they cry easily and are hard to settle; and they often seem negative about everything.

A third pattern is the "slow to warm up child," who is initially apprehensive and tense in new situations but, when given a chance to adapt, usually does so.

Elements of Temperament

The landmark research of Thomas and Chess described nine elements that constitute a child's temperament:

1. **Activity level:** Some babies seem to lie placidly most of the time. Others seem to be constantly in motion, their arms and legs usually moving one way or another.
2. **Distractibility:** Some infants can tune in to the task at hand and more or less ignore distractions. Others are easily distracted by a different activity.
3. **Intensity:** Some babies react much more strongly to a stimulus. For example, if they are upset or frightened, their cries seem louder and more shrill, and they persist for an unduly long period of time. It can be real work to settle these babies.
4. **Regularity:** Some babies establish routines for sleeping and feeding quite readily. You can tell without too much effort when they are likely to nap or nurse. Others seem to have no predictable schedule at all.

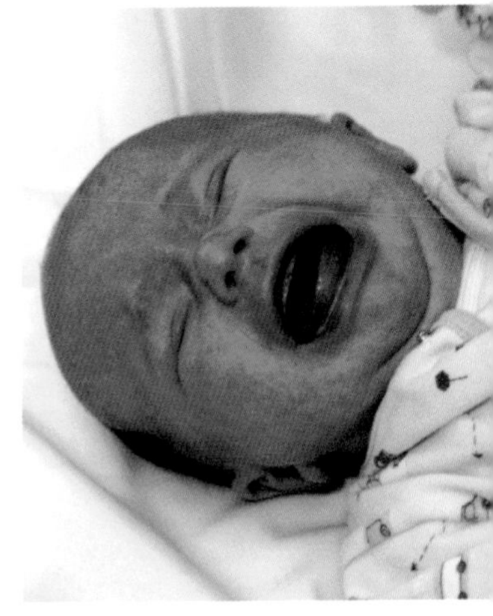

5. **Sensory threshold:** Some babies respond much more strongly to sound, sight, and taste than others.
6. **Reaction to new situations:** Some babies appear apprehensive in the presence of strangers or when placed in a new situation. Others seem relaxed in a strange environment.
7. **Adaptability:** Some children readily adjust to change and transitions; others don't.
8. **Persistence:** Some children are able to stay focused and persevere with the task at hand more than others.
9. **Mood:** Some infants seem serious, very negative, and dour. Others are constantly smiling and babbling contentedly. Most babies are somewhere in between these extremes.

HOW TO: Parent the Difficult Child

Clearly, parenting an "easy baby" is less exhausting and less frustrating than caring for a "difficult child." You did not choose your baby's temperament, but you must learn to deal with it. Here are some helpful tips:

- **Remember, it's not your fault.** Temperament is innate: you did nothing wrong. You are not a worse or better parent than the mother of that smiling baby sitting next to you in your parenting group.
- **Be consistent.** Try to identify his behavior patterns and routines, to the extent that they exist, then try to solidify these routines with consistency.
- **Take a break.** Parenting 24 hours a day can be exhausting. Schedule time for yourself each day. A fitness class, a coffee date with a friend — anything will do.
- **Get out of the house.** Taking the baby for a walk with another new parent is a lot more enjoyable than going alone. Enroll in parenting groups or infant gym classes for your sake as well as the baby's.
- **Share the load.** Chances are that Grandma would love to get a little more involved with the baby. Let her!
- **Cherish the good moments.** Somewhere in your memory bank, store the fact that the intense, determined infant often grows up to be the most successful adult.

Playtime

Despite what baby toy companies would have you believe, the most important equipment for playing with your baby is you! Babies love to be close to their parents. Your baby will be most interested in your face and voice, especially during his early months. During this period, your baby will spend most of his playtime listening and looking. As his development progresses, he will begin to interact with his environment and become more interested in touching, feeling, and mouthing objects. And as he becomes upright and eventually mobile, his interests will evolve.

Months 2 to 3

Your baby is not yet on the move and cannot talk or show you the toys he prefers. How are you supposed to play with him? Think about what stage of development your baby is at — it will guide you in your interaction and play. Follow your instincts and have fun!

Smiling

Babies usually start to smile by 6 weeks of age. Try smiling at your baby when he is alert, and look for that rewarding smile back! Teach him to interact by responding with a delighted sound or a soft touch when he smiles at you.

Talking

Your baby now enjoys listening to voices and is beginning to coo and make sounds. Encourage him by looking at him and slowly repeating similar sounds. Watch him watch your mouth with interest. Of course, there is no need to limit your speech to "baby talk." Talk as you would normally. Tell him what you are doing as you go about your day. These habits will all contribute to him learning about language and about you.

Cuddling, Rocking, and Singing Songs

These activities will be fun for your baby and may have a calming or soothing effect. Choose lullabies and nursery rhymes, such as "Twinkle, Twinkle, Little Star" and "Rock-A-Bye Baby."

Sitting Up

As your baby's head control begins to improve, you can set him down in different positions, with assistance, providing him with a new perspective on the world. Prop him up in a sitting position or gently raise him horizontally into the air, like an airplane.

KEY POINT

Be sure to take into account your baby's stage of development and choose activities and toys appropriate for his abilities.

DID YOU KNOW?

SAFE PLAY

At this stage, your baby's head control is still developing, so make sure you are with him during tummy time and other activities. If he falls asleep, place him on his back. Babies at this stage cannot grasp and move objects. Make sure your baby is always in a safe position, with his head and face unobstructed and away from soft blankets or toys that could interfere with his breathing. Toys should be soft, without sharp edges or small detachable parts.

Tickling

Now that your baby is smiling more and even beginning to laugh, play tickle games by establishing an association between a rhyme and a final tickle. He is enjoying learning about different sensations, so touch him softly, move his legs in a bicycling motion if he enjoys it, or try blowing softly on his toes. Find sensations he enjoys — you will be delighted by his response to them.

GUIDE TO: The Best Toys

There are many expenses involved in having children, but toys and play equipment do not need to use up your resources. A couple of bright rattles and a soft toy are nice to have, along with a mobile for your baby's crib. Otherwise, all your baby needs is a loving parent and a nurturing environment. Given that they are rarely used for more than a few months, toys can be borrowed from friends. Garage sales are another good source of toys, particularly for older infants.

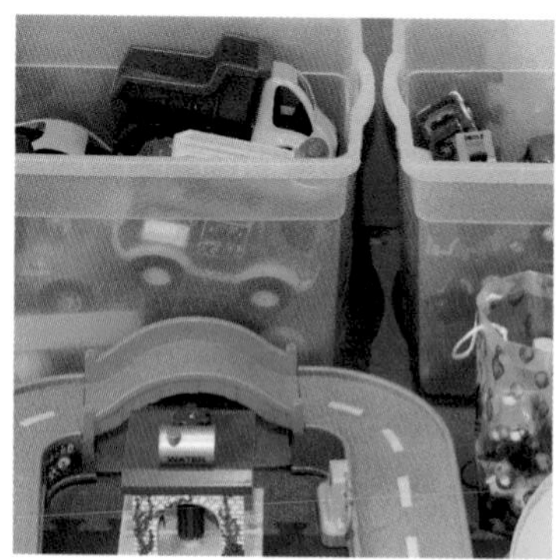

Rattles and Mobiles

You will likely notice that your baby intently regards his surroundings and has begun to follow objects. Babies enjoy looking at bold black and white patterns, as well as bright colors. With your baby lying on his back, show him some bright toys or rattles, moving them up and down and from side to side. Move the toy slowly up away from his face, toward the ceiling. He might begin to reach for the object, but don't expect him to successfully grab it at first. In time, if you place a rattle in your baby's hand, he will learn to grasp it and eventually give it a shake. He'll be delighted with the sounds he is helping to make, and may even reward you with a smile!

Other ways to stimulate your child visually include hanging a mobile above his crib or putting black and white or brightly colored pictures on the ceiling above his change table.

Activity Mats and Swings

Other popular items include seats that gently rock, in which the baby is harnessed securely; activity mats with toys hanging from above; and swings, which babies often find soothing. By no means are all of these big-ticket items essential. It is most practical to borrow them from friends or purchase them second-hand, as your baby may decide he is not a "swinger" or doesn't particularly like the seat. Even if he does like them, he will soon outgrow them.

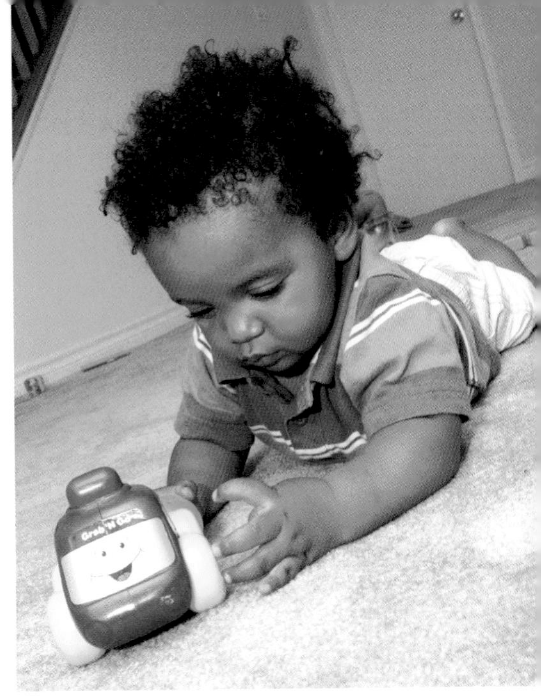

Months 4 to 6

This is a very exciting time in your baby's life. He is still an infant, and is not yet mobile, but he is becoming increasingly interactive and fun. Playing with your baby will both stimulate his development and bring you tremendous joy.

Continue to introduce your baby to the world around him. Many babies look with wide-eyed wonder at the bustle on the street or the produce in the grocery store. Talk to your baby about what he is looking at, encouraging his natural curiosity. Make a habit of describing what you are doing and seeing as you go about your daily activities.

Your baby's head and trunk control is increasingly strong, so he may be able to play sitting upright, with your support, as he gets closer to 6 months old. If you have a breast-feeding pillow, it can be used as a convenient support to prop him up. Otherwise, just use regular pillows.

Continue to place your baby on his tummy regularly. He'll soon be able to lift up his head and chest, which will make it a more comfortable position in which to look around and play.

Word Games

Your baby will vocalize more during this stage of development. Around 4 months, you may notice that when you make a cooing sound or talk to your baby softly, he responds with a sound back. With another sound from you, he may again respond. He is learning the basics of conversation!

As he continues to develop, he will start to play with sounds. If you make a funny noise, such as blowing a raspberry, you may get a laugh from him, and he may try to imitate you. Through this lively interaction, you are teaching him the basics of imitating sounds — an important skill that will help him learn to talk. As he starts to babble, around 6 months of age, he will enjoy hearing you imitate his sounds. Continue to talk to him as you go about your everyday activities. The sound of your voice and the words he hears will help him continue to learn basic language skills.

DID YOU KNOW?

PLAYPENS

A playpen can provide a safe environment for an infant, but remember that it needs to meet safety standards. It should be sturdy. The slats should be close together, and mesh should have small openings. Don't put anything inside that could be used to help an older infant climb out. Your baby needs to be out and about, exploring his environment, so use the playpen for short periods at a time.

Tickling Games

Tickling games are even more fun now, as your little one learns to anticipate your play. Wiggle your fingers and say, "I'm going to get you" or "Here I come," getting closer and closer until you end in a tickle and giggle! Although many babies find this fun, some find it too much or can engage in this stimulating play only very briefly. Watch for your baby's cues and choose activities he enjoys, ending when he has had enough.

DID YOU KNOW?

TASTING THE WORLD

By now your baby is likely putting everything (including his own toes) in his mouth. This is his way of exploring new things; provided the objects are safe, this behavior should not be discouraged.

Action Songs

As he becomes more interested in his environment, your baby will love watching and listening to action songs. Try "Itsy Bitsy Spider" or "I'm a Little Teapot." Nursery songs, as well as children's rhymes, are often a favorite with children of this age.

Mirror Games

Babies generally become increasingly social during these months. They begin to recognize people, and they enjoy admiring themselves in the mirror. Many toys incorporate mirrors for babies to gaze at, but your bathroom mirror works just as well. Hold your baby while you stand in front of a mirror, wave, and talk to him. He will likely be delighted at seeing both his reflection and yours.

Age-Appropriate Toys

Apart from toys to grasp, chew, and roll, very little additional equipment is needed. Give your baby colorful toys that he can easily grasp, pick up, and eventually transfer between his hands. Rattles, hard plastic rings that loop together, or plastic balls with holes for him to grasp are good examples of appropriate toys for this age. If your baby is teething, hard plastic teething rings can be cooled in the refrigerator and make good toys for your baby to play with and chew on.

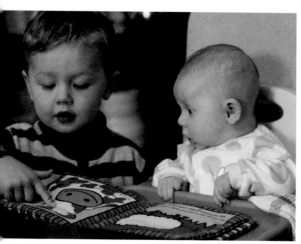

Provide a variety of textures for your little one to explore. Introduce soft toys or stuffed animals, as well as objects with different gentle textures. Soft toys can get dusty and collect germs, so make sure they are washable. Brightly colored cloth or board books with a single picture on each page are appropriate at this stage. Activity centers with colorful, bright, textured toys to touch, spin, and look at are often a favorite.

Try to find toys that produce gentle musical noises as opposed to loud, irritating sirens. If the noises are really obnoxious, the batteries can always be removed as a last resort!

As you take your baby out of the home more, you may choose some toys that can be safely fastened to the stroller or car seat.

Exersaucers

Your baby may be ready to play in an exersaucer during this time. An exersaucer is a stationary ring that surrounds the baby and holds stimulating toys to keep him entertained. Ensure that it is used as recommended at the appropriate height (this can usually be adjusted for your baby's growth over the coming months). Exersaucers should be used for short periods at a time — usually no more than 20 minutes. Keep the exersaucer away from dangers such as hanging appliance cords or stairs.

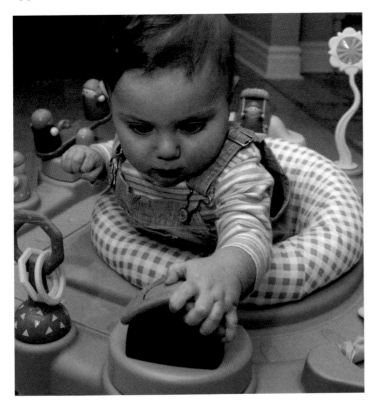

DID YOU KNOW?

BABY WALKERS

Baby walkers have been banned in many countries, including Canada, because they are extremely dangerous for babies. Many children are injured every year while in a walker, usually under the close supervision of a parent. Infants in a walker can move more than 3 feet (1 m) in 1 second, and children have rolled down stairs, gotten burned, and even drowned. If you are given an old baby walker, get rid of it immediately!

Frequently Asked Questions

Should we be worried that our baby's weight percentile is less than the percentile for her length?

Weight loss, when it occurs, is worrisome. But don't be too concerned if your baby is growing steadily along a certain weight percentile, even if it is less than her percentile for length.

Our breast-fed 5-month-old seems a little chubby. What should we do about it?

Nothing. Even though obese children often become overweight as adults, obese infants — especially those who are breast-fed — don't necessarily become overweight children. Infants tend to slim down once they become mobile. Breast-feeding on demand is the preferred form of infant nutrition. Restricting nursing time is seldom a good idea.

Can I safely fly with a 2- to 6-month-old baby?

Yes, but use some common sense:

- Give yourself lots of extra time to get to the airport. You'll need it.
- Change the baby shortly before boarding, then take advantage of early boarding opportunities.
- To reduce earache, encourage your baby to suck on something, such as a pacifier or bottle, during ascent and descent.

My 6-month-old baby loves to stand and bounce when I support her, but I worry that it will cause bowed legs. Will it?

No need for worry. Standing supported at this age is good exercise, not a cause of bowed legs.

Is something wrong if my 5-month-old still isn't rolling over?

A baby's developmental milestones are individualized. Some skills will come earlier than usual, while others might appear later. It is the overall developmental pattern you should pay attention to. Now that babies are placed on their backs to sleep, many seem in no rush to roll over by 4 or 5 months.

Why does my daughter put everything in her mouth?

Infants love to explore the world around them. Often, they use more than sight and sound to do so: they also use their mouth and tongue to explore shape and texture. The real trick lies in ensuring that what goes in her mouth is safe.

Can I "spoil" my baby at this age?

Being responsive to your baby is just meeting his needs. At some point, children must learn that the world doesn't revolve around them, but this is not that time.

When my 5-month-old daughter sees her grandfather, she often cries. It is very upsetting for everyone. What can we do?

By this age, infants have developed the ability to differentiate caregivers from strangers. Some babies are quite cautious and react poorly even to people who love them. Allow your baby time to warm up to new situations and individuals who are not regular caregivers. Frequent exposure and shared pleasurable moments will ultimately forge positive bonds.

My baby and I love to spend time outside. But sunscreens are not recommended until 6 months, so what can I do to protect him?

Keep going out, if that is what you both enjoy; just avoid the peak hours of sun exposure, between 10 a.m. and 2 p.m. Use clothes and umbrellas that block ultraviolet rays. And if it comes down to a choice between sunburn and sunblock, choose sunblock. Products that contain microparticles of titanium dioxide are unlikely to cause problems, even in young babies.

At what age can we use a framed backpack-style baby carrier?

Most backpack-style carriers can be used once a baby turns 6 months of age. The baby should have good head control and trunk strength.

My baby's eyes still seem crossed. Is that normal for a 4-month-old?

In the first month or two, an infant's gaze may not be coordinated, or "conjugate." By 4 months, though, the eyes should not be turning in. Have your doctor look into the problem.

My 5-month-old still spits up. Will it ever stop?

Spitting up, or gastroesophageal reflux, is still normal at this age. You don't need to worry unless your baby repeatedly chokes or wheezes with feeds, is gaining weight very poorly, or seems irritable when swallowing (which suggests that the esophagus is inflamed). In over 90% of infants, gastroesophageal reflux resolves before the first birthday.

Are exersaucers bad for my baby's development?

No. And, for busy parents, they can be very useful. Exersaucers are commonly used, safe, practical aids to help you entertain your baby. As long as you use them in moderation and do not leave your baby in one for hours or unattended, they will not have any negative effects on him.

CHAPTER 7

Introducing Solid Food

KEY POINT

Solid foods are sometimes started as early as 4 or 5 months by parents who simply can't wait to begin. However, introducing solid food long before 6 months or long after 6 months is not recommended.

Remarkable changes occur in a baby's diet during the first year of life. The tiny newborn who once fed exclusively on breast milk or formula has, by the age of 1 year, become a regular member of the family, sitting in a high chair, joining in mealtime activities, and eating more or less the same meal as everyone else.

Parents view the introduction of solid food to their baby's diet as a significant milestone. But introducing solids to your baby can be confusing. When solid foods should be offered, what foods should be offered, how much food should be offered, and in what sequence — these are questions you will need to answer in consultation with your health-care providers, but there are some general guidelines you can follow.

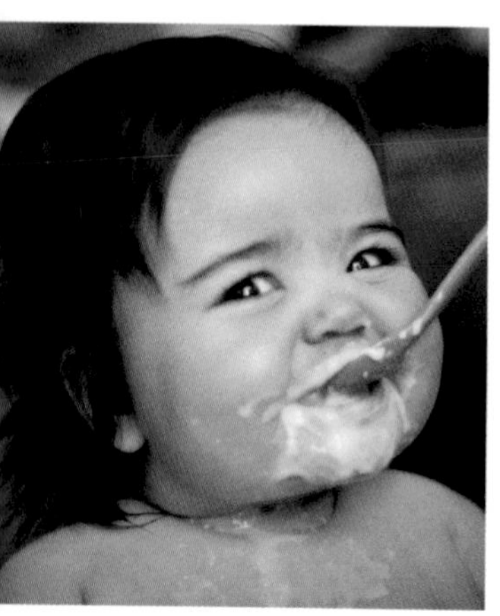

When to Start

No healthy, thriving baby, whether breast- or formula-fed, requires solid food during the first 6 months of life. In fact, the World Health Organization, the American Academy of Pediatrics, and the Canadian Paediatric Society recommend that babies be breast-fed exclusively for the first 6 months.

Not Before 4 Months

There are several good reasons not to start solids earlier than 4 months of age. First, solid foods simply aren't needed until then. Breast milk or infant formula provides ample nutrition. Second, your baby may be neurologically too immature to be fed solids safely. An infant may still have her primitive extrusion reflex, which helps with nursing but interferes with solid foods moving easily from the front of the mouth to the back of the throat. Third, even supported, it is difficult for a very young baby to be placed properly in a sitting position before 4 months. Fourth, a baby's gut is still quite immature before 4 months of age; as a result, digestion of some of the protein in solid foods may be incomplete, which can lead to a food allergy in some cases.

KEY POINT

Although you may have heard that giving your baby cereal at night will help her sleep, there is no scientific evidence to suggest that this is true.

Not Long After 6 Months

There are equally good reasons not to wait longer than 6 months before starting solids. Though breast milk or infant formula will continue to be your baby's primary source of nutrition between 6 months and 1 year, neither provides the amount of iron she requires. In addition, if solids are not introduced before your child reaches 9 months, she might decide that drinking fluids is much easier than eating solids and resist being introduced to textured foods.

When She's Ready to Eat

In addition to these medical considerations, your baby will be ready to eat solid foods when specific physical and developmental milestones are achieved:

- She can sit with support and hold her head up nicely.
- She shows an interest in your food and may even begin to try to feed herself.
- After breast-feeding or bottle-feeding, she seems to want more.
- She wants to feed more often.
- She opens her mouth to put toys in, and if you put a small spoon in, she can keep her tongue low, as opposed to pushing the spoon out.
- She uses her tongue to help move food into the mouth and shows signs of a chewing motion.

DID YOU KNOW?

IRON NEEDS

Increasingly, medical science is recognizing how essential iron is for infant learning and development. Up until about 6 months of age, your baby benefits from iron stores acquired in the womb. At 6 months, however, those stores are running out, and your baby needs supplementation from solid foods in her diet — over and above what breast milk or formula provide.

Feeding Principles

Though common sense and parenting instincts should always prevail when you're feeding your child, here are a few general principles to follow:

- Decide *what* your child eats and let her determine *how much* she eats.
- Choose healthy foods. Save chocolates and deep-fried foods for special treats. Select natural products, free of excessive preservatives or sugar substitutes.
- Allow your baby to feel in control of her mealtime. Let her open her mouth by herself before you try to place food in it. Let her explore the food, touch the spoon, or use her fingers to put food in her mouth. Let her decide on the pace of things and, when she seems to have had enough, stop feeding her, even if some food is left on her plate.
- Introduce your baby to a wide variety of foods, but hold off on honey until she is at least 1 year of age because of the risk of botulism infection.
- Avoid adding salt or sugar to your baby's food. (The same advice should probably apply to everyone in the family.) Instead, you can season food gently with common herbs and spices, such as rosemary, thyme, sage, or even mild curry, to allow your baby to become accustomed to your family's tastes.

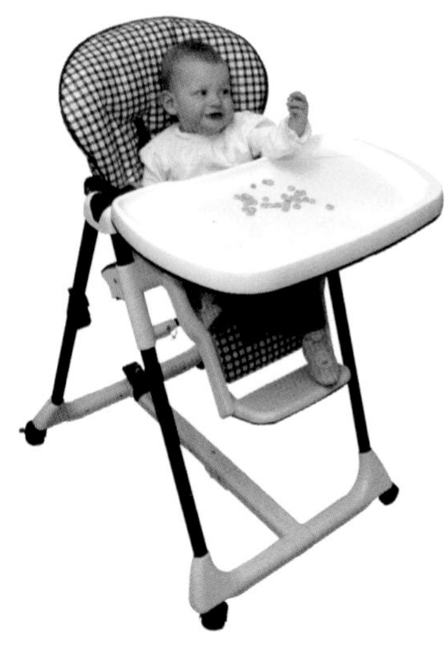

Feeding Equipment

Feeding is no exception to all of the other milestones your baby reaches — it is accompanied by a deluge of information from marketing companies about the equipment you must buy. In truth, there are only a few items you need to get started.

High Chairs

Initially, you may choose to feed your baby in any infant seat in which she is upright and secure. Ultimately, you will need a proper high chair for your baby's comfort and safety. Features of a good high chair include a comfortable seat that supports your baby in an upright position and strong straps with a proper buckled harness.

Other features to consider are wheels, if you plan to move the high chair around your kitchen, height adjustments to allow for your baby's growth, and a removable tray that can be easily cleaned. It is useful if the tray has a lip to limit how much food ends up on the floor — which will inevitably happen!

DID YOU KNOW?

PORTABLE HIGH CHAIRS

Depending on your lifestyle, you may wish to invest in a portable high chair. Made of plastic, with straps that allow them to fasten to a regular chair and a tray that snaps on and off, these are relatively inexpensive.

Bowls

When your baby begins solids, no special bowls are required because you are feeding her. As she develops and begins to feed herself — either with her fingers or a spoon — your need for plastic bowls will depend on your tolerance for broken dishes! Inexpensive plastic bowls or plates are a practical option.

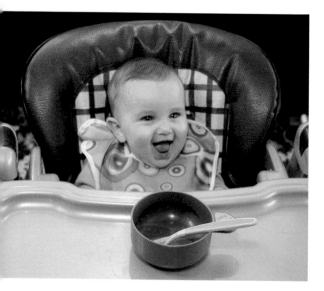

Spoons

Plastic infant spoons are a nice way to start, and several can be purchased in one package. Their flexible handles and shallow heads make them ideal for little mouths. Older babies or toddlers can graduate to slightly deeper spoons or little forks, but make sure the handle is small enough for their hands to grasp.

Bibs

Starting solids will be — and should be — a messy experience. Your baby will explore each new texture with her hands and her mouth as she determines her likes and dislikes while learning to eat with increasing independence. Needless to say, bibs are a must! Either cloth or plastic is acceptable, though you will probably find the plastic ones more convenient for wiping off with soapy water between meals. Most fasten around the neck with either a snap or Velcro, and bigger ones will cover most of your baby's front.

Bottles and "Sippy" Cups

Unless babies are nursed exclusively, most will use a bottle at some point. Unfortunately, babies quickly learn to love the bottle itself, and not just what's inside! Remember not to let your baby take milk or juice to bed.

An alternative option is to introduce a "sippy" cup, a plastic cup with a lid and a valve system in place to prevent liquids from spilling out when the cup is turned upside down. Though you may associate their use with toddlers, there is no reason they can't be introduced to a baby. The valve dictates that a certain degree of "suck" be generated for your baby to get the fluid out, but babies as young as 6 months can begin to get the hang of it. Though babies learn to love sippy cups, they don't tend to be as "addictive" as the bottle, which makes volume control and transitions easier.

There are lots of ways to introduce sippy cups. Try offering water from the cup early on, then gradually offer milk or formula from the cup one feed at a time. If you've nursed your baby exclusively for several months, you could even go directly to the cup (in addition to continued nursing) for water and eventually milk, skipping the bottle stage altogether. Even if your baby doesn't understand right away that the cup is for drinking, let her play with it and watch you drink from a cup. She will certainly work it out in time!

What Foods to Start With

Iron-fortified cereals have long been recommended as the first complementary foods to introduce, but iron-rich meat and meat alternatives are now recognized as another ideal starter food.

DID YOU KNOW?

PORTABLE FOOD

You will want to be prepared to carry food for your baby with you, whether you're traveling far away or just to a friend's house for lunch. Food is easily carried about in plastic containers with tops. If your baby is eating infant cereal, just pour the desired amount of powder into the bowl and add the liquid when it's time to eat. Baby food in jars is easily portable; if you're making your own, simply place an appropriate portion in a container. There are lots of portable healthy snacking options for children who are exploring finger foods.

KEY POINT

Never let your baby take a bottle of milk or juice to bed! Bottles in bed promote tooth decay.

KEY POINT

At 6 months your baby is not getting enough iron from breast milk or formula alone, so her first solid foods, whether cereals, meats or meat alternatives, should be iron-rich.

KEY POINT

Wait about 3 days after introducing a new food before you try another, so you can observe how well each is tolerated.

Your baby's transition to solid foods should be gradual. Introduce one new food at a time and wait a few days before introducing the next. That way, you can easily identify the cause of any reactions or allergies, if they occur.

Your ultimate goal is to be feeding your infant from the four basic food groups — cereals and grain products, meat and alternatives, vegetables and fruit, and milk and dairy products — over the course of the day, creating a well-balanced diet of carbohydrates, protein, and fats that is rich in vitamins and minerals.

Cereals

Single-grain, iron-fortified baby cereal is an excellent starter food. Infant cereals are bought as a powder, which can be mixed with expressed breast milk, formula, or water to the desired consistency — be sure to read the label for which of these is required. Many commercial brands are available, and there is no best one to choose, as they are all iron-fortified. Most people begin with a rice cereal, as rice is the grain least likely to produce an allergic reaction. Once your baby has adjusted to eating rice cereal by spoon, she can try other single-grain cereals, such as oatmeal or barley. After she has tried each of the single-grain cereals, you may introduce her to mixed cereals.

HOW TO: Prepare Infant Cereal

1. Initially, mix cereal to the consistency of thin porridge, then gradually thicken it to whatever density your baby seems to prefer, which in most cases is a soft mush.
2. Serve cereal from a bowl, using an infant spoon.
3. Never feed your baby cereal from a bottle; the texture will be diluted, and this method can interfere with the development of her feeding skills.
4. Start with 2 to 3 teaspoons (10 to 15 mL) of cereal, given once daily; as your baby catches on, gradually progress to whatever amount seems to interest and satisfy her, usually 2 to 4 tablespoons (30 to 60 mL) twice a day. These volumes are just a guide.
5. Feed your infant as much or as little as she wants to eat. Some babies take longer than others to adjust to textures. Your baby may take very little one day and surprise you with higher volumes the next. The most important marker – not just with cereals, but with your infant's nutrition in general – is that she is growing and developing normally, not the number of teaspoons she takes at each feed.

Meat and Alternatives

You can also introduce a source of protein as one of your baby's first solids. Examples include red meat, poultry, fish, eggs, beans, or tofu. At this stage, your baby's food should be puréed. Meats can be puréed in a food processor, while eggs and soft tofu are easily mashed. Commercially prepared protein foods for this age group are all in purée form.

These new foods can be given at the same feed as cereal or offered separately as a third or even fourth feed.

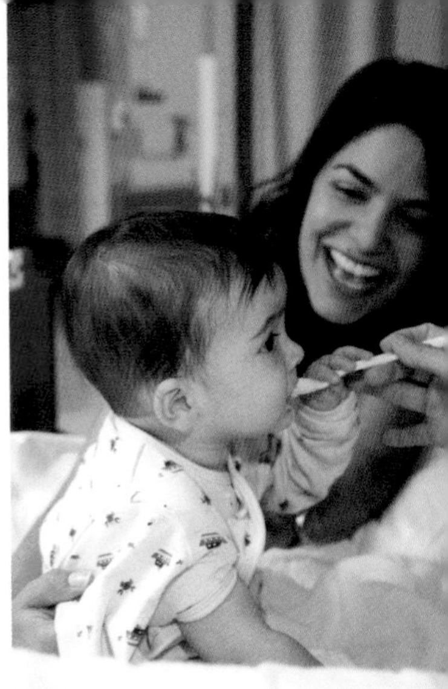

Vegetables and Fruits

Once your baby is accustomed to infant cereals, usually between 6 and 7 months of age, it is time to add cooked and puréed vegetables and fruits. Yellow, green, and orange vegetables, as well as all varieties of fruit, are appropriate. Common choices include carrots, squash, green peas, pears, applesauce, and bananas, but anything goes.

There is no "right" order in which to introduce these foods, though many people suggest serving vegetables before fruits so that your baby doesn't become accustomed to sweet flavors and reject her veggies. There is no science, however, behind this largely theoretical suggestion. Offer a variety of vegetables and fruits and enjoy watching your baby experiment with new tastes and textures.

Begin by offering vegetables or fruit twice a day, in addition to infant cereal and meat/meat alternatives. At the beginning, the consistency should be a smooth purée because your baby is just learning about different textures and doesn't yet have the ability to chew. Introduce each new flavor with a positive attitude. Your baby will pick up on your feelings about what you're providing, so try not to influence her with your own likes and dislikes. Eventually, your baby will determine her own favorites and express dislike for some foods. When this happens, wait a few days or longer, then try the food again — you may be pleasantly surprised as your baby adjusts to the new flavor or texture.

KEY POINT

As you introduce solid foods, don't be concerned if the color and consistency of your baby's stools change. What you see in the diaper will vary depending on her diet each day, and it is not unusual for small undigested pieces of fruit or vegetables to appear in the stool. This is normal, as long as your baby is growing well. What goes in is generally more important than what comes out.

Milk and Dairy Products

Dairy products can also be introduced around this time to provide an important source of fat, protein, and calcium. Be sure to give your baby full-fat options until she is at least 2 years old — fat is vital for proper brain development.

Plain yogurt, grated cheese, and cottage cheese are excellent choices. Homogenized cow's milk can be introduced at 9 months, but it is better to wait until your baby is a year old. Before then, she is at risk of iron deficiency because cow's milk is low in iron, can displace iron-rich foods, and inhibits absorption of iron. Continue to feed her breast milk or infant formula until you make the switch to cow's milk. Of course, breast milk may be continued even longer, if desired.

Introducing Solid Foods

FOODS	FROM 6 TO 9 MONTHS	FROM 9 TO 12 MONTHS
Breast milk	Nursing on demand	Nursing on demand
Iron-fortified infant formula	On demand, about 3–5 feedings every 24 hours	On demand, about 3–4 feedings every 24 hours
Iron-fortified infant cereal	Offer 2–3 tbsp (30–45 mL) twice daily	Offer 2–3 tbsp (30–45 mL) twice daily
Other grain products	Introduce other grain products, such as dry toast or unsalted crackers	Introduce other plain grains such as bread, rice, and pasta, 8–10 tbsp (120–150 mL) daily
Meat and alternatives	Offer puréed cooked meat, fish, chicken, tofu, beans, or egg, 1–3 tbsp (15–45 mL) daily	Offer minced or diced cooked meat, fish, chicken, tofu, beans or egg, 3–4 tbsp (45–60 mL) daily
Vegetables	Offer puréed cooked vegetables (yellow, green, and orange), progressing to soft mashed vegetables, 4–6 tbsp (60–90 mL) daily	Offer mashed or diced cooked vegetables, 6–10 tbsp (90–150 mL) daily
Fruit	Offer puréed cooked fruits or very ripe mashed fruit (such as bananas), 6–7 tbsp (90–105 mL) daily	Offer soft fresh fruit, peeled, seeded and diced; diced canned fruit packed in water; or juice, 7–10 tbsp (105–150 mL) daily
Milk and dairy products	Offer plain yogurt (3.25% MF or higher), cottage cheese, or grated hard cheese, 1–2 tsp (15–30 mL) daily	Introduce whole (3.25% MF) cow's milk, moving from a bottle to a cup. Continue with full-fat or high-fat plain yogurt, cottage cheese, or grated hard cheese, 1–2 tbsp (15–30 mL) daily

Adapted with permission from Daina Kalnins and Joanne Saab, *Better Baby Food, Second Edition* (Toronto: Robert Rose, 2008).

Food Allergies

Food allergies occur when a person's immune system reacts to a food protein that the body identifies as "foreign." Symptoms range from severe anaphylaxis (facial swelling, hives, and difficulty breathing, requiring immediate medical attention) to non-specific symptoms such as abdominal pain, vomiting and diarrhea, wheezing, or skin rash. Although extremely rare, anaphylaxis can sometimes occur as the first sign of a food allergy.

True allergies are different from food intolerance, in which symptoms occur in response to a particular food but are not due to an immune reaction.

While people of any age can develop allergies, children's immature digestive systems make them more susceptible. Some common allergies, such as those to cow's milk protein or eggs, are outgrown by the majority of children. If you are worried that your baby may be at increased risk of allergies, discuss this with your health-care provider.

Common Food Allergies

In infants, the most common food allergens are cow's milk and eggs. An allergy to the protein in cow's milk can be seen in 2% to 5% of formula-fed infants, usually starting in the first month. Symptoms may include blood in the stool, diarrhea or vomiting, irritability, and poor weight gain. Even breast-fed babies whose mothers consume dairy products can develop symptoms.

Many children, particularly those who react to milk and eggs, will "outgrow" their allergies; in the case of cow's milk, 80% to 90% of infants who are allergic to it will tolerate it by the age of 3 years.

Peanut, nut, and shellfish allergies generally become evident in older children as they become exposed to them. Sensitivity to peanuts, nuts, and shellfish tend to persist.

Treating Food Allergies

Food allergies are best managed by avoiding specific allergens. To manage cow's milk allergy, for example, breast-feeding mothers are often asked to try a dairy-free diet, while formula-fed babies are usually switched to a special hypoallergenic formula.

Infants who exhibit signs of a food allergy beyond a mild skin reaction should be seen by a physician. They will be

KEY POINT

The recommendations regarding introduction of potential food allergens, such as fish and eggs, have changed in recent years. Delaying their introduction is not advised, even for babies who may be at increased risk of allergy or atopy (eczema or asthma). These foods can generally be introduced after 6 months of age.

DID YOU KNOW?

ACIDIC FRUITS

Acidic fruits (berries, tomatoes, citrus) can sometimes cause a reddish skin rash around the mouth; this does not usually lead to a true allergic reaction.

referred to a specialist, who will perform various tests, such as skin prick testing, to determine the allergen.

Anaphylaxis is a medical emergency. If your baby's mouth or throat shows signs of swelling, she is having trouble breathing, and you notice a change in alertness, call 911 so she can be taken to the emergency department of your local hospital immediately.

If your child is diagnosed with a food allergy, caregivers may be instructed on the use of an epinephrine auto-injector, such as an EpiPen, to be used in case of a significant reaction. The specialist may also recommend that your child wear a MedicAlert information bracelet.

HOW TO: Minimize the Risk of Allergies

In the past, parents were advised to hold off on introducing highly allergenic foods, such as eggs, nuts and fish, until children were older than 1 year. Despite this precaution, the prevalence of food allergies in children seems to be increasing and is estimated to currently affect 5% of children under 5 years in the United States. Recent studies suggest that earlier introduction of potentially allergenic foods may actually *prevent* food allergy. The theory is that, if babies are not exposed to them early enough, their immune systems will treat these foods as foreign substances and attack them, resulting in a food allergy.

The following general recommendations are based on the existing studies and current expert consensus opinion, but may change as more evidence from ongoing trials becomes available:

1. Do not avoid highly allergenic foods during pregnancy.
2. Do not avoid highly allergenic foods during breast-feeding unless your baby has shown signs of allergy to a particular food.
3. Breast-feed exclusively for at least 4 months; this seems to reduce the risk of allergies.
4. Introduce solids around 6 months and no earlier than 4 months.
5. Introduce single-ingredient foods first, no faster than one new food every 3 to 5 days.
6. Once a few typical solids are tolerated (cereals, meats, vegetables, fruits), introduce potentially allergenic foods and watch carefully for any allergic reactions.
7. If you have an older child with a peanut allergy, ask your child's health-care provider whether to expose your baby to peanut butter at home or under the supervision of a medical professional. In this scenario, your baby's risk of also having a peanut allergy has been estimated at 7%.

Mealtimes

Initially, it's better to respond to your baby's signals than to a clock. Begin by offering cereal just once a day, and progress to twice daily as your baby gets the hang of things. This affords her twice the opportunity to learn that the pasty stuff on the spoon is actually satisfying. Remember that your baby's primary source of nutrition remains breast milk or formula, so these cereal feedings should not interfere with nursing or the bottle.

Hunger Response

There are no "rules" about what time of day solids should be given. However, many parents find it easiest to give the earliest morning feed as breast milk or formula rather than cereal — especially for breast-feeding mothers who need to relieve overnight engorgement. Cereal can then be offered when your baby expects her second feed of the day. Generally, it's best to offer cereal at the beginning of the meal and then "top it up" with breast milk or formula. That way, the baby is a little hungrier and thus more motivated to experiment with new tastes and textures.

A Regular Schedule

As your baby is introduced to more food groups, her feedings will begin to resemble meals in terms of the variety offered and satisfaction achieved. As your schedule allows and your baby demands, two feedings a day will gradually become three meals. When your baby is older still, morning and afternoon snacks will be incorporated.

Though a strict schedule is not necessary, it is never too early to introduce positive eating habits by establishing a routine. Offer the first meal, for example, when the rest of the family is up and ready for their breakfast; enjoying breakfast together is a wonderful start to any day. Provide your baby with supper when everybody is gathered again at the end of the day. That way, mealtime can be a family event.

From Purées to Finger Food

Preparing food for your baby at this stage is an exciting experimental process of introducing new textures, colors, and flavors. Your baby will quickly let you know her likes and dislikes. Have fun preparing her favorite foods.

DID YOU KNOW?

SETTLING HUNGER PANGS

When she's first starting solids, if your hungry infant cries persistently because she hasn't yet learned to appreciate cereal, you can settle her and her "hunger pangs" by offering the breast or bottle for a brief initial period. When she has settled, retry the cereal.

KEY POINT

Your baby's energy needs are unpredictable. Trust that she will know what she requires. The amount of food consumed day to day, feed to feed, and baby to baby will vary. That's normal. Offer your baby the amount of food she seems to crave, but don't force her to take more than she wants. Conversely, don't withhold food if she appears hungry. Long before she has words, your baby will communicate very clearly when she's hungry or full!

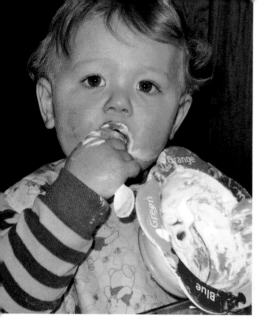

Homemade vs. Store-Bought Purées

Whether you make your own baby food or buy commercially prepared puréed food is up to you. Homemade foods are simple to prepare and allow for more variety at a lower cost; however, they can be time-consuming to make. Store-bought foods are manufactured under stringent hygiene conditions and are equally nutritious.

Give your baby the opportunity to appreciate the natural flavors of fruits and vegetables, without added sugar or salt. In a few months, when she is eating a broader range of foods, feel free to experiment with mild seasonings and spices.

HOW TO: Prepare Homemade Baby Food

- Wash fruits and vegetables carefully. Peel and remove stems and ends.
- Cook, bake, or grill meats; do not fry them. Be sure to remove any skin, bone, or gristle.
- Mash or purée most food to the consistency of applesauce. A food processor or blender makes puréeing fruits and vegetables easy, and is also ideal for beans and meats. Fresh or frozen vegetables can be boiled or steamed until soft. Place the cooked produce in the food processor or blender and purée. You'll need to add a little water – usually between 1 and 3 tablespoons (15 and 45 mL), depending on the vegetable – to reach the desired consistency. Meat and poultry require more water and a longer processing time.
- Some foods don't require any special preparation. Examples include bananas, avocados, and soft tofu, all of which are naturally soft and can be mashed as required with the back of a spoon.
- Prepare batches of food for several meals.
- Store freshly prepared purées in the refrigerator or freezer. To freeze purées, first pour them into ice cube trays. (Some specialty baby stores sell trays with lids specifically for this purpose.) Once the cubes are frozen, transfer them to freezer bags. Be sure to write the contents and date on each of the freezer bags – sweet potatoes and squash can look very similar! Thaw the cubes as needed. Cubes are an easy way to measure out portions.
- Try using food "nets." Some babies enjoy sucking on larger pieces of fruit using nets designed for this purpose. Pieces of melon, for example, are placed inside the net so that your baby can suck the juice from the fruit without the risk of choking on larger pieces.

Finger Foods

While every baby is different, by the age of 8 or 9 months, most infants are ready to try more textured finger foods (foods that can be held in their hands). Children who are ready for finger foods have probably been introduced to all of the major food groups and have developed the skills to sit alone, pick up food with their fingers, bring it to their mouth, and chew with some degree of success. These newly acquired skills represent quite an accomplishment, but don't expect this process to be neat — just enjoy the feeding experience, however messy.

If you're not sure whether your child is ready for finger foods, offer a trial of soft food, such as grated cheese or small pieces of very soft fruit, and watch to make sure she doesn't gag or choke. Take note of whether she enjoys this new experience. If she is not yet ready, continue with purées for another few weeks, then try again.

Continue to feed your child cereal as a source of iron, though you may decrease cereal feeding from twice to once a day as her diet expands to include other iron-rich foods such as red meat and leafy green vegetables. Breast milk or formula feedings should also continue, though their quantity will naturally decrease.

Safety First and Last

Choking is a significant hazard when solid foods are introduced. Babies like to explore with their hands and mouth and may inadvertently swallow food before you have mashed it for them. Signs of choking include coughing, gagging, and wheezing. Consider taking an infant CPR course so you'll be prepared should this situation arise.

Reducing the Risk of Choking on Solid Foods

- Never leave a feeding baby unattended.
- Don't allow your baby to crawl or walk with food in her mouth.
- Feed your baby in a high chair.
- Carefully examine fish for bones, even tiny ones.
- Cut all foods into small pieces. Foods such as hot dog slices or whole grapes can completely plug the throat or windpipe. Cut them lengthways into quarters to be safe.

KEY POINT

When you do make the transition from purées to finger food, be sure to do so gradually. It will take your baby time to adjust to new textures and the work involved in eating finger foods, so her diet is best supplemented with ongoing offerings of a well-balanced diet of purées.

DID YOU KNOW?

HONEY

Before you know it, your baby will be enjoying a balanced and varied diet. Although variety is the spice of life, some foods are better introduced a little later in your child's life. Wait until your baby is at least a year old before you give her honey. The bacterium *Clostridium botulinum* may contaminate unpasteurized honey, posing a theoretical risk of contracting botulism. Botulism is a very serious disease that results in severe swallowing difficulties, muscle weakness, and constipation.

- Avoid foods that can crumble or shred and be aspirated into the lungs, such as whole nuts and whole raw carrots. Serve carrots cooked or grate raw carrots to prevent choking.
- Avoid hard candies, cough drops, popcorn, peanuts, nuts, seeds, gum, thick spreads, and any other food you're not sure your baby can handle.

GUIDE TO: Appropriate Finger Foods

As with purées, continue to offer your baby a variety of foods, both to satisfy her tastes and interest and for their diverse nutritional value. Ensure that food is soft enough to be easily mashed by your baby's gums and that it is cut into small pieces — generally no larger than $\frac{1}{4}$ to $\frac{1}{2}$ inch (0.5 to 1 cm).

Following are some common examples of foods to try, but the options are endless, so be creative!

- Peeled soft fruit, such as bananas, ripe cantaloupe, pears, or peaches, cut into bite-size pieces
- Soft cheese, or hard cheese that is grated or thinly sliced
- Cooked tender meat, ground or cut into small chunks
- Fish, soft tofu, mashed beans, or egg (all are good sources of protein)
- Mashed or diced cooked vegetables (favorites include green beans, spinach, carrots, potatoes, and tomatoes)
- Soft bread, oat rings, or crackers that easily dissolve (try them out in your own mouth)
- Cooked short pasta

Meat is often the most difficult food for infants to adjust to because it can be difficult to chew. Many recipes can be made with ground meat, including meatloaf or lasagna, which can then be cut into small pieces. Try softening meat with gravy or tomato sauce.

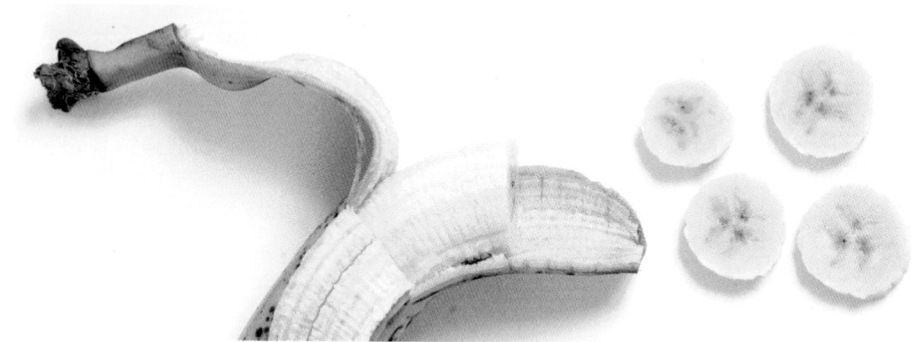

Frequently Asked Questions

Should I feed my baby or allow her to try feeding herself?

When you first introduce your baby to solids, she will not have the developmental capability or the desire to feed herself. At this stage and for the first few months, she will rely on you to feed her with a spoon. Between 8 and 12 months, she will begin to use her fingers to feed herself, initially by grasping soft cookies or crackers. Give her the opportunity to feed herself at least some of the time. One tactic is to feed her for the first part of the meal, ensuring that a good portion of the food winds up in her mouth, and allow her some independence as she finishes off.

Your baby will also learn from you as you use utensils to eat. By all means, offer her a soft spoon to explore. She'll initially play with it, but by 11 months of age or so, she may impress you by picking it up by the handle. Though she likely won't feed herself exclusively until several months down the road, these early opportunities to explore and learn are invaluable. Ignore the mess — and be sure to offer praise and encouragement as success is achieved!

My 9-month-old son insists on feeding himself. He's not very good at it, and I worry that he won't get enough to eat. What should I do?

Don't worry — his desire for independence will not result in starvation. Hunger inevitably trumps autonomy. By this age, your son has probably developed a pincer grasp and finds picking up food by himself quite enjoyable. It's okay for him to experiment with textured foods, such as pieces of cooked macaroni, well-cooked ground meats, and mashed bananas or potatoes. He won't be able to use a spoon yet, but will probably let you feed him his favorite purées or, at least, let you help him use the spoon.

How much should I feed my baby?

Most people's food intake varies from day to day and often from meal to meal. Babies are no exception. Some infants also seem to eat more than others. Don't worry if your nephew gulps down everything in sight, while your own child seems quite picky. Rather than sticking to a strict feeding regimen, it's best to let your baby's appetite determine how much she should consume.

How often should I feed my baby?

Because mealtime is a great family time, try to make breakfast, lunch, and dinner an important part of your baby's routine between 9 and 12 months. Around this time, morning and afternoon snacks are also introduced to satisfy your baby's hunger between meals. Snacks add an important nutritional component to your baby's diet, provided that healthy snacks are offered. Depending on your baby's nursing or bottle routine, his snack may be finished off with some breast milk or formula.

When can I introduce cow's milk?

As your baby's nutritional requirements are increasingly met by her solid food intake, the quantity of breast milk or formula she drinks will gradually decrease. While you may choose to nurse your baby for longer than a year, formula may be replaced with homogenized cow's milk by 1 year of age. This transition is not recommended prior to 9 months, and closer to 12 months is preferred to ensure that your baby's gut is mature enough to tolerate cow's milk protein and that she is consuming a sufficient quantity of iron-rich foods.

When you do introduce your baby to cow's milk, remember that, while it is an excellent source of calcium, it does not contain the same quantity of iron or other nutrients found in infant formula. You may choose to transition your baby gradually, continuing to offer some formula, as well as infant cereal and meat.

It is also important to limit your baby's milk intake to 16 to 20 ounces (480 to 600 mL) per day. More than that will put her at risk for iron deficiency, due to possible microscopic blood loss from the gut. Babies also have a tendency to fill up on milk in place of nutritious solid food; decrease the chance of this happening by offering milk during or after mealtime, not before.

Should I give my baby water?

While newborns do not need water, by 6 months of age it is appropriate to offer your baby water to quench her thirst. Of course, water has no nutritional value, so your baby shouldn't fill up on water prior to mealtimes. Offering it with meals, however, or on a hot day, is a good idea. In terms of quantity, there is no guideline as to how much water your baby needs. Let him be the judge.

My baby still gets up at night. Will feeding him cereal at bedtime help him sleep through the night?

No. Cereals aren't sedatives. Babies sleep through the night when they are ready to do so.

What about juices?

Many parents view fruit juices as a "natural" food that can be harmlessly consumed by babies without concern or limit. Wrong. Fruit juices are loaded with sugar and can cause many problems. A bottle of juice in the crib at bedtime may soothe your baby, but it can also produce serious tooth decay. Undiluted juice may cause cramps or even diarrhea. Fruit juices can also kill a baby's appetite for more nutritious foods, including milk. Of course, this doesn't mean an infant should never be offered apple or grape juice. Just remember that moderation is the key. Here are some helpful guidelines to consider:

- Encourage your baby to drink water instead of juice to quench her thirst.
- Introduce fruit juice no earlier than 6 months of age (some say to wait until 1 year).
- Dilute fruit juices with equal amounts of water to reduce unnecessary calorie intake. Unsweetened apple juice, for example, contains 124 calories in every 8-ounce (250 mL) bottle.
- Limit the amount of juice a child receives daily to 4 to 6 ounces (120 to 180 mL).

CHAPTER 8

Your Baby's Months 7 to 12

Now the fun really begins! During the second half of infancy, your little one becomes eager to explore, is mobile, and loves to interact and converse with you. He is acquiring new skills daily, and just as you think you have him all figured out, he changes. His independence becomes apparent, and along with it, the need for appropriate strategies to deal with various behaviors. Separation anxiety also peaks around this time. At this stage, being read to, playing games with you, and exploring the world are some of his favorite activities.

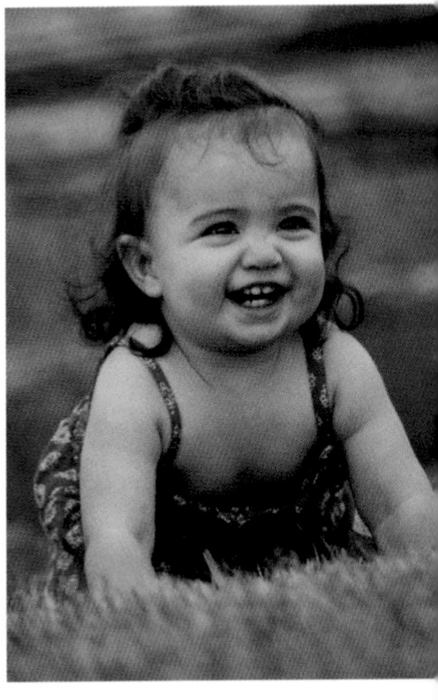

Still Growing and Developing

As your baby progresses through this period, his growth continues in weight, height, and head size, but at about half the rate of the first 6 months. Infants at this age continue to develop motor skills rapidly. As a result, they become much more interactive and playful.

Growth Curves: 7 to 12 Months

Growth measurements will typically be taken two to three times during this period, usually at around 9 months and again at the 1-year visit. By 1 year of age, an average infant has tripled his birth weight, has grown by one-quarter of his initial length, and has gained about 4 inches (10 cm) in head circumference.

Your child's growth should be followed carefully as he transitions to eating solid foods, to ensure that he continues to meet his nutritional requirements. It is expected that he will continue to follow along the curves on his growth chart.

Some parents fear they are overfeeding their babies. Excessive chubbiness usually becomes less of an issue when the baby starts to become more active and increases in height. It is not appropriate to make dietary adjustments in the first year of life — for example, cutting down on fats or carbohydrates — because your baby needs these to fuel his growth and development. As he gets older, there will be other ways that you can encourage the development of healthy eating habits.

DID YOU KNOW?

HEIGHT PREDICTION

Some parents become overly concerned about the short stature and chubbiness of their children at this age. The best predictor of ultimate height is the midpoint between the mother's and father's height. The vast majority of children in the developed world will reach this potential, even those with rather odd eating habits in the early years.

Development Milestones: 7 to 9 Months

During his second 6 months of life, your baby will achieve several major milestones, and his newfound abilities will open up a whole new world of fun and exploration.

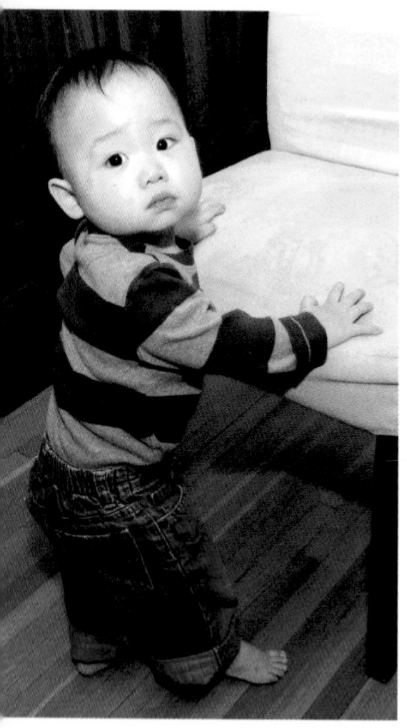

Sitting and Holding

By 7 months, most babies are able to sit securely and hold objects in their hands at the same time — quite an accomplishment!

Crawling

Most infants of this age are able to crawl, with varying degrees of dexterity. Some begin with "commando crawling," dragging their body by pulling ahead of them with alternating arms. Others progress straight to their hands and knees. Some babies never crawl.

Standing

Many infants are able to pull themselves up to a standing position by 9 months of age. Once they are up, they may have a hard time getting back down. If you haven't already done so, this is definitely the time to move things from coffee tables and night tables up higher! Make sure there are no sharp edges to bump into. At this stage, when mobility far exceeds agility, many little falls are likely to occur.

KEY POINT

Whatever your baby picks up will inevitably make its way into his mouth, so make sure little objects are not left lying around, especially by older brothers and sisters, whose toys are likely full of choking hazards.

Picking Up Small Objects

Growing control of hands and fingers leads to attempts to pick up smaller objects, initially by trapping them between the baby finger and palm, and gradually moving toward a thumb and index finger pincer grasp. At this stage, your baby may start to hand a toy to an adult, but has trouble letting go.

Communicating

At this age, your child will continue babbling and should be using a number of different sounds. He will imitate funny sounds you make and laugh at them. He is capable of shouting and is not afraid to practice this new ability.

Throwing Objects

Your baby is now aware that objects out of view are still there and will look for a toy that has fallen or rolled away.

In fact, he is likely to practice this newfound wisdom by repeatedly throwing objects, such as food, spoons, and dishes, from his high chair and expecting you to pick them up. This is not done with the intent of driving you crazy — it is a normal stage of development!

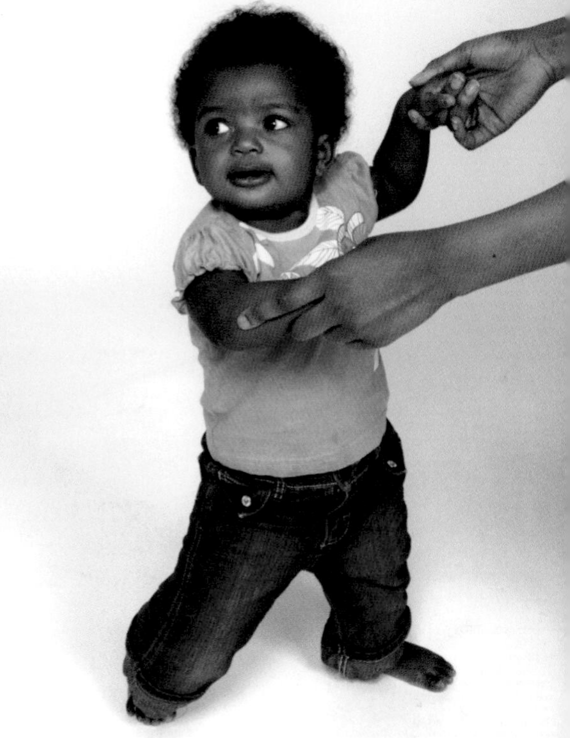

Development Milestones: 10 to 12 Months

Toward the end of the first year of life, most babies become mobile — crawling, rolling, creeping, cruising, and ultimately walking. His mobility is going to change things dramatically for everyone concerned. If you haven't already fully childproofed your home, don't wait any longer!

Cruising

At 10 months, many infants start to cruise: walking along while holding on to furniture with both hands. Soon this will progress to walking with his hands held by an adult, and just when you think your back can't take it anymore, he will take those exciting first steps. Don't worry if he's not quite there yet — most babies generally start walking between 12 and 15 months.

Picking Up, Pointing, and Drawing

By this time, your baby will be able to pick up small objects, such as Cheerios, fluff, and dust specks, with his precise thumb and index finger pincer grasp. He is starting to point to objects and is able to hold a bottle or cup. Around 1 year of age, infants can hold a crayon in one fist to make marks on paper.

Speaking

Your baby's babbling is becoming more purposeful. By 1 year of age, many babies are able to use "Dada" and "Mama" with meaning — sweet music to the ears of parents who have been waiting for this moment for some time! By 12 months, your child will generally know and respond to his name.

> **DID YOU KNOW?**
>
> **INTERACTING WITH YOUR BABY**
>
> As your baby gains more understanding of the world around him, he will become increasingly interactive. Peekaboo and tickle games engage his attention. He will start to clap his hands and wave goodbye, new skills that bring with them a host of new clapping and bye-bye games.

Playtime

Play is the work of babies! Playing with your baby is an important part of parenting. Your baby learns to communicate and interact by playing. Play is also essential for your baby's brain development. It is a time for you and your baby to enjoy interacting with each other, without distractions. By showing your baby that you enjoy your time with him, you create a relationship that gives him a sense of security and forms the foundation for his relationships with others.

Reading to Your Baby

Reading to your baby promotes intimacy and bonding, and stimulates acquisition of language and intellectual skills. In the latter half of the first year, babies start to enjoy reading with their parents. Innumerable books are available for you and your baby to enjoy. Incorporate reading into your baby's daily routine, and you will set the stage for a lifelong love of reading.

Most babies enjoy hearing the same story over and over again. This is normal — children learn through repetition. Books with nursery rhymes and those with familiar objects for naming are great. Songs and rhymes make words easier to remember, making the language come alive.

As they get closer to 1 year of age, babies are able to hold a book and turn the pages. Start to point to things and name them. If your baby loses interest or is easily distracted, skip to a favorite page or put the book down and try again later.

KEY POINT

There are many ways to encourage and initiate reading with your baby. Being a good role model is the best place to start. If your baby sees you reading regularly, especially if you hold him close while you are reading, he will learn early on that reading is a positive behavior.

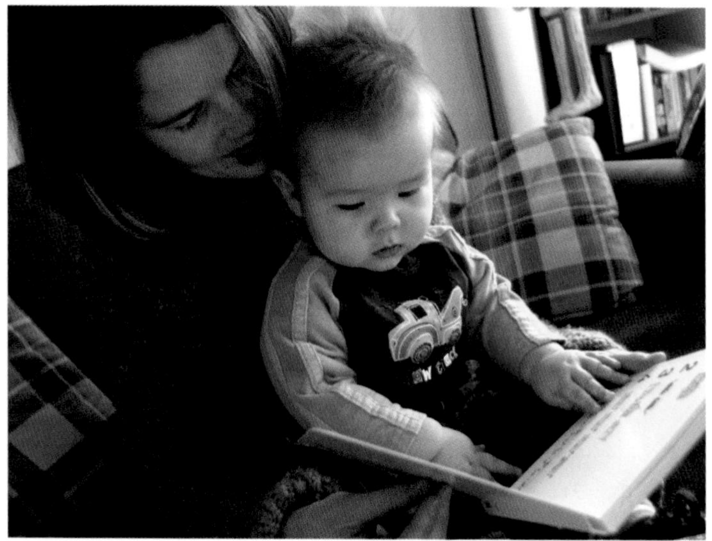

Age-Appropriate Toys and Activities

As a result of your baby's rapidly developing skills, appropriate toys and activities change substantially from the predominantly sensory toys recommended for younger infants. Now he will begin to enjoy activities that involve moving, banging, pulling, squeezing, pouring, throwing, opening, closing, inserting, and removing.

- **Interactive games:** Your baby will start to engage in activities such as peekaboo, hiding and uncovering games, imitating sounds and actions, and a great, timeless favorite: baby drops the object, adult picks it up. Most children of this age love bath time and water activities. Your encouraging words, clapping, and enthusiastic "hurrays" as you interact will encourage your baby's play and build his confidence in his growing abilities.
- **Toys:** Stacking blocks, rings, or cups, objects that fit into each other, and pop-up boxes are very popular. Infants like to push and follow movable toys, such as large balls and cars. Some babies enjoy simple puzzles. Basic household items such as plastic cups, containers, and pots can provide hours of entertainment, learning opportunities, and noise!
- **Books:** Many 6- to 12-month-old children will start to develop a real interest in books. Simple, colorful illustrated books made of cloth, plastic, or cardboard are ideal, as many young children are able to manipulate the large, thick pages, and the books are relatively resistant to being torn, soaked, or chewed. Talk to your baby in simple language about the pictures in the book. Label objects and point to them. Choose books that have large pictures of other babies or familiar objects such as toys and animals, or books that illustrate familiar experiences, such as bath time or mealtime. Books with large flaps that lift up, uncovering an interesting picture underneath, are popular and encourage fine motor development.

DID YOU KNOW?

SCREEN TIME

The American Academy of Pediatrics and the Canadian Paediatric Society recommend no screen time for children under the age of 2. This includes tablets, phones, computers, and televisions. Even programs and games that claim to be educational should be avoided. Instead, read a book to your child, sing songs, or play a game. Experts agree that exposure to and interaction with real people is far more beneficial, both academically and socially.

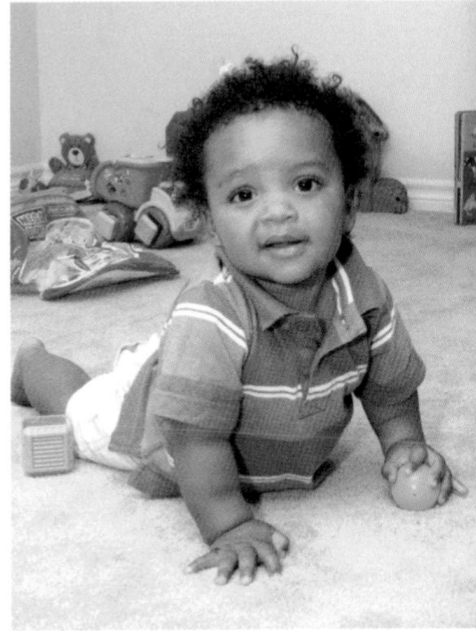

Disciplining Your Child

It may seem premature to start thinking about disciplining your baby at this age. However, by introducing your values and expectations early on, you can lay a solid foundation for your child's behavior for many years to come.

GUIDE TO: Safe Toys

Toy safety is paramount for babies, who have developed skills that allow for manipulation and motion but have no awareness of potential harm. Toy manufacturers in North America are required to follow stringent safety laws. For example, toys with small parts that could be a choking hazard are labeled as such. Be aware that toys made in other countries may not be as strictly regulated as those made in North America.

Keep these safety tips in mind when you buy toys for your baby:

- **Size:** Be sure the toy is too big to fit in a baby's mouth, ears, or nose.
- **Small parts:** Avoid toys with small parts that could choke your baby. Toys intended for older children may have dangerous small pieces, so pay attention to age recommendations.
- **Solid construction:** Test toys to be sure they are well constructed and will not break easily. Eyes and noses on soft toys should be sturdily fastened.
- **Sharp edges:** Avoid toys with sharp or pointed edges.
- **Safe materials:** Make sure toys are made from a safe material intended for small babies, and avoid items decorated with paint that may chip off — it may be toxic. Be sure any fabric used in making the toy is not flammable.
- **Hazards:** Avoid toys with strings or cords that pose a strangulation hazard. Never allow your child to play with balloons, which can cause choking and asphyxiation.
- **Batteries:** Ingestion of watch-type batteries is extremely dangerous. Make sure these are kept out of reach of inquisitive hands.
- **Cleanliness:** Be sure toys can be cleaned easily.
- **Packaging:** Safely dispose of all plastic wrappings and bags.

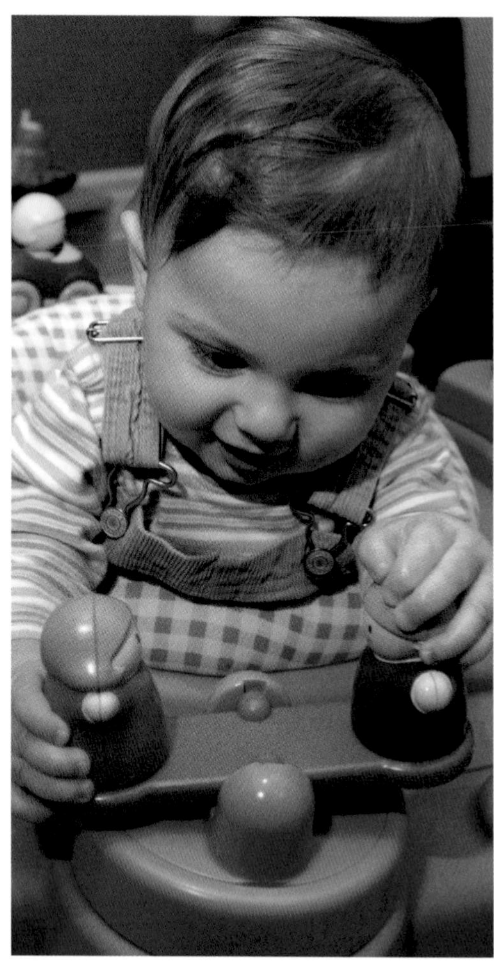

There are no absolute rules of discipline. Individual children have different temperaments, and parents have varying approaches, priorities, and expectations. So methods of discipline should be individualized. Caregivers should be consistent, so that it is clear to your baby what the limits are. Even very young children quickly figure out who can be easily manipulated to allow them to break the rules.

Appropriate Strategies

Time out and punishment are not appropriate strategies in the first year of life, but distraction, removal, and ignoring unwanted behaviors are useful techniques. For example, if your baby keeps pulling your hair, give him something else to play with or pull on. Alternatively, tie your hair up so that he cannot reach it. He will probably become bored with the game and move on to something more entertaining. Sometimes a firm "no," coupled with a negative facial expression, gets the message across very clearly. But remember, although we are all human, acting out of anger is not good parenting, no matter how tired or frustrated we feel. If anger, not teaching, drives your discipline, then it's time to get some help.

Safety

In this age group, safety is a major focus for discipline. Infants 7 to 12 months of age are very curious about the world around them. They reach and grab objects. When they become mobile, they seek to explore their environment. This curiosity is not matched with judgment and experience.

Children must be taught their limits and appropriate boundaries. Not only should you ensure that their environment is safe and provide close supervision, you must teach children safe behavior. If your child tries to grab something that is hot or fragile, firmly say "no," remove him from the object, and distract him by giving him something else to play with. If you are consistent, he will learn that some objects are not appropriate for him to play with.

Consideration for Others

It is not too early to begin teaching your baby to be considerate of others. If you are attending to the needs of an

KEY POINT

Discipline is most effective in an environment where a child feels comfortable and secure. In older children, negative consequences are sometimes necessary to reduce undesirable behavior; however, in infancy, positive reinforcement and encouragement are the most effective forms of discipline.

DID YOU KNOW?

DISCIPLINE DEFINED

Many people equate the term "discipline" with punishment. But discipline is not punishment. The word is derived from the Latin word for "teaching." According to the American Academy of Pediatrics, "discipline is a whole system of teaching based on a good relationship, praise, and instruction for the child on how to control his behavior. Punishment is negative; an unpleasant consequence for not doing something. Punishment should only be a very small part of discipline."

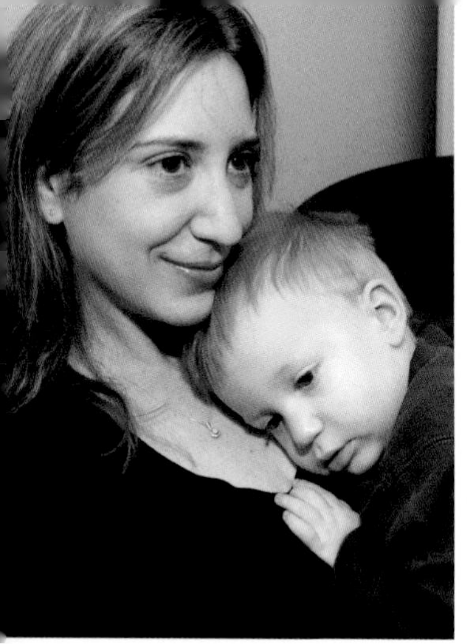

older brother or sister, it's okay to deal with the older child first. It's not necessary to drop everything and immediately respond to the baby. A gentle voice should reassure your infant that you will get to him as soon as you can.

What's Normal, After All

As babies grow older, they continue to develop their unique personalities. In so doing, they may exhibit several behaviors that appear unusual to you. The majority are normal and usually transient.

Separation Anxiety

Separation anxiety is a normal stage of development during which infants develop emotional discomfort and seem anxious when separated from familiar caregivers. The degree and duration of separation anxiety can vary tremendously between infants depending on their individual temperaments. Some babies develop separation anxiety at a few months of age, while others are always happy to be picked up and entertained by strangers. These are the extremes. Most infants develop some degree of separation anxiety around the age of 9 months, not only when you leave your baby with someone else but also when you try to put him down for the night.

Typically, separation anxiety lasts until about 2 years of age, although new experiences, such as starting school or going to camp, can precipitate separation anxiety in older children.

DID YOU KNOW?

OBJECT PERMANENCE

Separation anxiety should be seen as part of normal development as your baby develops a sense of object permanence and memory. Object permanence means that he knows you are still around even when he can't see you. For younger babies, out of sight is usually out of mind! The development of memory means that, when he sees the babysitter or sees you getting ready to go out, he remembers that this means you will not be there for him for a while. This is distressing to him.

Coping with Separation Anxiety

Having your baby cry every time you leave him can be very upsetting. Here are some strategies for alleviating separation anxiety:

- When possible, try to leave your baby with a consistent caregiver, with whom he will become accustomed to spending time.
- Have the babysitter come over a while before you need to leave — it gives her a chance to engage the baby in a fun activity while you are still there.
- You may think it is easier to sneak out and avoid a scene, but for some infants, this can be confusing and anxiety-provoking. He may start to cling to you to make sure you

don't disappear again. An alternative plan is to give him a little advance warning that you are going out and a big hug and kiss as you are leaving, reassuring him that you will be back and will see him later.

KEY POINT

Most infants settle quite easily once their parents are out of earshot.

Breath-Holding Spells

Sometimes a child, seemingly in response to being upset or frustrated, stops breathing and turns dusky or very pale. He may actually lose consciousness for a moment or two. In extreme cases, some twitching or jerking of the limbs may occur. The episodes usually last for about a minute — it only seems like much longer! It's pretty scary stuff, but, in fact, breath-holding spells are both common and benign.

Breath-holding episodes occur in about 5% of children, most often between the age of 1 and 4 years, but sometimes in infants as young as 6 months. Rarely, a painful experience or sudden startle can initiate a breath-holding spell. These spells are not harmful and require no specific treatment. Nor are they associated with neurological or psychological problems. Still, because they fear triggering a spell, parents may stop setting reasonable behavior limits for their child — which is not a good idea.

Confirm with your doctor that any losses of consciousness are indeed consistent with breath-holding spells. Once you are sure that breath-holding is the cause, hasten the disappearance of this behavior by ignoring it and not giving it positive reinforcement.

DID YOU KNOW?

PLAYING WITH THEIR OWN HAIR

Some babies like to stroke, twirl, and play with their own hair, especially when they are tired. This is usually a comforting, soothing habit, and is not of concern.

Breath-Holding Red Flags

Advise your doctor if your baby's breath-holding episodes have any of the following characteristics or you think there may be something else wrong:

- They are not precipitated by crying, frustration, or pain.
- They last longer than 1 minute.
- They occur before the age of 6 months.

Rhythmic Movements

Some babies engage in rhythmic movements such as head banging, head rolling, or body rocking. These repetitive motions may continue for several minutes and usually occur when the child is going to sleep. Most experts believe that they are self-comforting movements. This behavior generally commences around the age of 6 months and resolves around 2 years of age. If the child is otherwise healthy and developing normally, there is no cause for concern. However, if your child has any other unusual behaviors or developmental delays, consult your doctor.

Exploring the Genitals

KEY POINT

When children get older, teach them that playing with their genitals should be done in a private place.

Many infants discover their genitals during the second 6 months of life, usually in the bathtub or during diaper changes. They also discover that it feels good to stimulate them by touching them. You may notice that your little boy sometimes gets erections. Some little girls rub their vaginal areas against fixed objects, such as the strap of the car seat or even table legs. A form of masturbation, this self-stimulation is completely normal behavior in children of all ages. There is no reason to be concerned.

Biting

The primary teeth usually start to erupt during the second 6 months of life, and your baby will subsequently learn to bite and chew. Many infants will take the opportunity to bite down on anything that comes close to their mouths, including Mom's breast and other people's fingers, cheeks, noses, and ears. As the teeth get bigger and more numerous, this can be very painful for the victim.

KEY POINT

Despite your misgivings about your baby's biting, he is not being angry or hostile. Biting is a normal part of experimental behavior, and is usually a transient phenomenon.

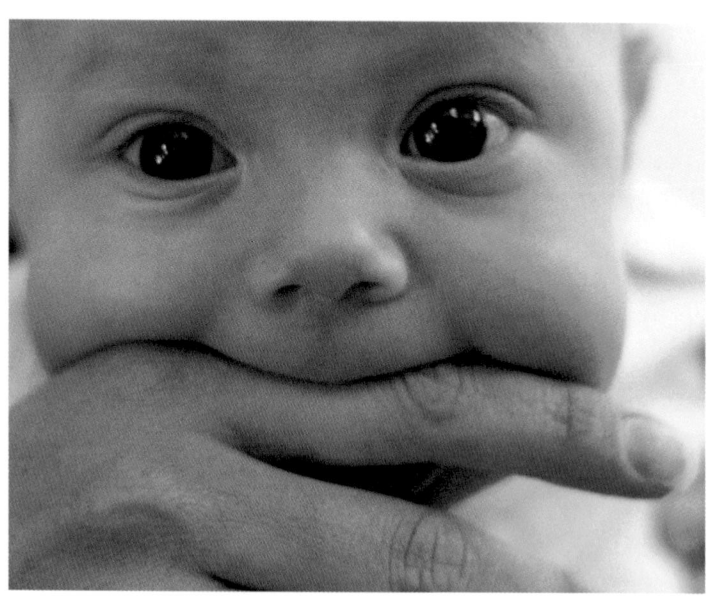

Preventing Excessive Biting

Your baby needs to learn that biting is not acceptable. Biting is sometimes reinforced by the reaction it provokes: it is natural to startle and react with facial and verbal expressions when you are bitten. Try not to respond dramatically.

The most effective response is to calmly remove your baby from the body part he has bitten, firmly say "no," then move on to another activity to distract him. If you do this repeatedly and consistently, your baby will learn not to bite.

Tooth Grinding

Tooth grinding, also called bruxism, occurs in up to half of normal infants, usually once the upper and lower incisors have erupted. It is not clear why babies grind their teeth — it is probably because "they are there" and the infants enjoy the sound or sensation. Tooth grinding is most frequent at night, and can be very annoying or worrisome for parents. Fortunately, it is a habit that wanes with time, and it does not cause permanent damage. The best treatment is to ignore it.

KEY POINT

Late eruption of teeth does not interfere with learning to chew and eat solid foods; babies can manage very well with their gums.

Teething Time

Your child will eventually have 20 primary, or "baby," teeth — 10 on the bottom and 10 on the top. The order in which teeth erupt can vary, but the bottom central teeth, called the lower incisors, are usually the first to emerge. Often, teeth appear in pairs rather than one at a time.

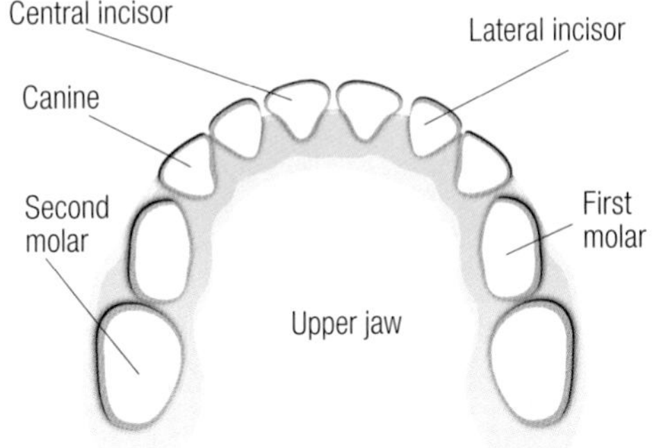

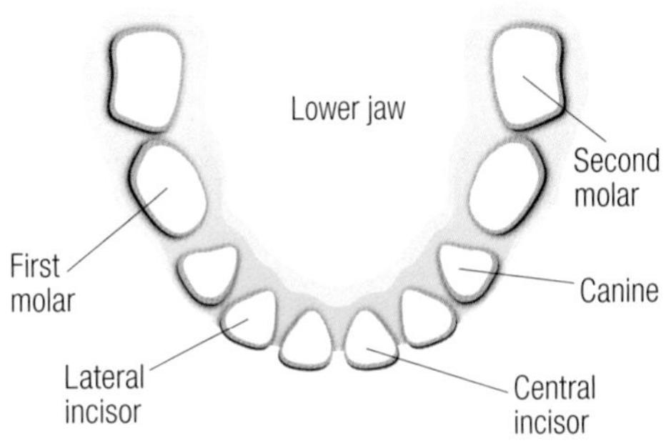

First Teeth

The age at which a baby's teeth first erupt is extremely variable. On average, the first tooth emerges at about 7 months, but some babies are born with a few teeth in place, while others don't get their first teeth until after their first birthday.

If no teeth have erupted, no intervention is required until at least the first birthday. Thereafter, your health-care provider may decide to check for a hormone or vitamin deficiency.

Normal Eruption Pattern

	TOOTH	ERUPTION	FALLS OUT
Upper jaw	central incisor	7 to 12 months	6 to 8 years
	lateral incisor	9 to 13 months	7 to 8 years
	canine	16 to 22 months	10 to 12 years
	first molar	13 to 19 months	9 to 11 years
	second molar	25 to 33 months	10 to 12 years
Lower jaw	central incisor	6 to 10 months	6 to 8 years
	lateral incisor	7 to 16 months	7 to 8 years
	canine	16 to 23 months	9 to 12 years
	first molar	12 to 18 months	9 to 11 years
	second molar	20 to 31 months	10 to 12 years

Teething Symptoms

Teething has been blamed for a myriad of symptoms, including drooling, diarrhea, facial rashes, fever, congestion, sleep problems, and irritability. But teething is not necessarily the culprit behind all or any of these problems. The first teeth tend to arrive at the same time that your baby's antibodies (which crossed over through the placenta before birth) are beginning to wane, resulting in an increase in infections, including ear infections, colds, and gastroenteritis. Teething is often coincidental and not the cause of a given problem.

DID YOU KNOW?

HOMEOPATHIC REMEDIES

Homeopathic teething remedies do not always clearly state what they contain and are not subject to rigorous testing. There have been reports of toxicity, including lead and mercury poisoning, so these remedies should either be avoided or be used with caution.

Treating Teething Symptoms

Most infants tolerate teething very well. If your baby appears to be in pain, consider these do's and don'ts of teething.

Do's

- Do massage the gum with a clean finger.
- Do let your baby bite on a cold wet washcloth or refrigerated teething ring.
- Do try teething biscuits.

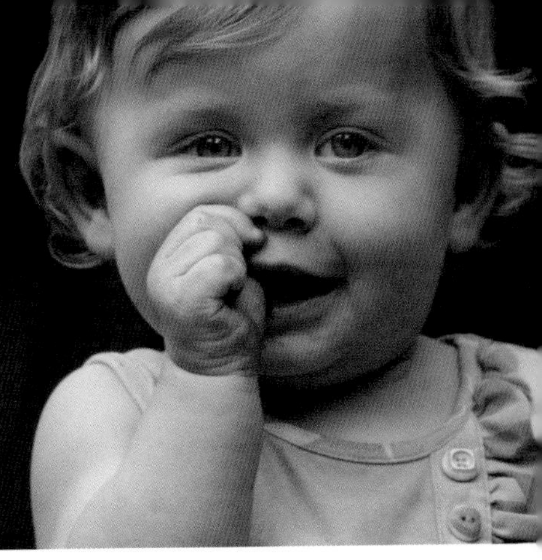

- Occasionally do give a dose of acetaminophen or ibuprofen for the discomfort (but do not do so on a regular basis).

Don'ts

- Don't use teething gels (there are potential side effects, and they're not very effective).
- Don't use homeopathic teething remedies (they are potentially toxic).
- Don't allow biting on cut-up vegetables, such as carrot sticks (they're a choking hazard).
- Don't feed your baby honey (there's a risk of botulism).
- Don't give your baby alcohol!
- Don't place teething rings around your baby's neck (there's a risk of strangulation).

Dental Caries (Cavities)

Dental caries refers to the presence of one or more decayed teeth (with or without a cavity), missing teeth (due to decay), or filled tooth surfaces in any primary tooth. Caries are caused by bacteria, which break down the sugars we eat. This process, in turn, produces acid. The acid destroys the minerals that make up our teeth. The enamel of a baby's tooth is immature and susceptible to breakdown. Untreated, decay can lead to infection and pain. This can spread to the face or other parts of the body and make your child very unwell. Decay and infection can also spread to the jaw bone and damage the development of permanent teeth.

One of the most common causes of dental caries in young children is going to bed regularly with a bottle of milk or sugar-containing fluid.

Brushing Your Baby's Teeth

Dentists recommend starting to clean the teeth as soon as they erupt. Starting early helps to ensure good dental hygiene and habits. Teeth cleaning should become part of the bedtime routine.

You can gently brush your baby's teeth with a small, soft toothbrush or wipe the teeth and gums with a clean, moist piece of gauze. Toothpaste is not necessary at this age. If you choose to use it, it should not contain fluoride. Another useful option is a small device that looks like a soft thimble, made of rubber with soft bristles on one side.

KEY POINT

Dental decay can start in the first year of life. Good oral hygiene is essential, even for a young infant without teeth.

DID YOU KNOW?

VISITING THE DENTIST

The first visit to the dentist should occur within 6 months of the first tooth eruption or when your child is 12 months old, whichever comes first. The dentist can determine if the cleaning you are doing at home is working. Going to the dentist at a young age will help make your child more comfortable in the dentist's office and help to identify and fix any dental problems early.

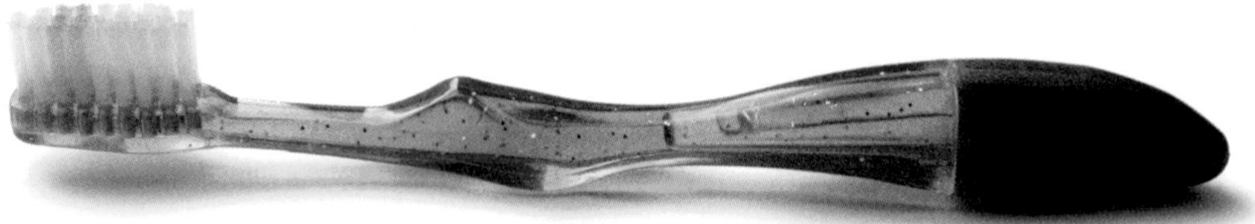

HOW TO: Prevent Dental Caries

Dental caries is the most common disease in children worldwide. Taking good care of your baby's primary teeth is very important because they are the precursors for his permanent teeth. Here are some tips for preventing cavities:

- Babies and young children should not be allowed to sleep with a bottle containing milk or juice in their mouths. Even small amounts of sugar-containing fluids constantly dripping into the mouth will result in dental decay. This is known as bottle caries. It may also be seen in babies who breast-feed frequently at night, usually those who co-sleep and nurse intermittently and often.
- Fruit juices – even when diluted with water – should be avoided for as long as possible because the high sugar content promotes dental decay. Instead, give your baby fruit to eat and breast milk, formula, or water to drink.
- Teach your baby to drink from a cup before he reaches 1 year of age. This helps to get him away from the constant drip of sugary material (including milk!) onto the teeth from the bottle.
- Do not dip your baby's pacifier in anything sweet.
- Parents and pregnant women should practice careful dental hygiene to help prevent the spread of bacteria to their infant.

Outings

Going outside is now a true treat for parents and baby, but is still a bit complicated. A walk, run, or bicycle ride in your neighborhood should be part of your daily routine, unless, of course, the weather is extremely cold or excessively hot and humid. Always make sure to take a change of clothing, a snack, and a drink for your baby.

Clothing

In general, babies over 6 months do not need to be dressed much more warmly than adults and older children. Bear in mind, though, that if you are walking vigorously and your infant is sitting in a stroller, you are likely to feel warmer than he does. If it is cold outside, ensure that his head, ears, hands, and feet are covered. In wet or windy weather, transparent covers for the stroller provide good shelter from the elements. Stroller covers to protect your baby from the sun and mosquitoes are also available.

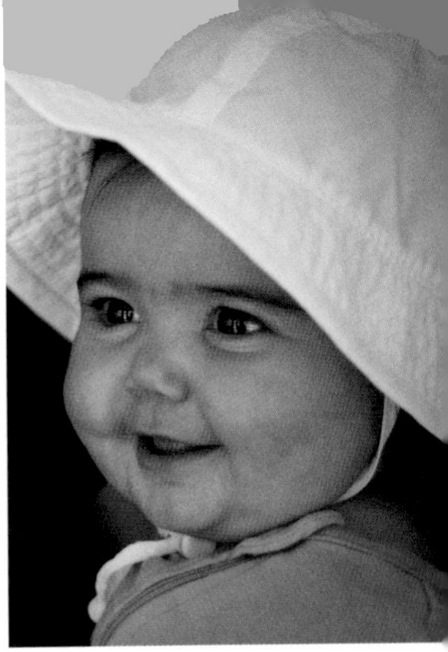

Sun Protection

Sun exposure during childhood is the greatest single cause of damage to people's skin. Sunburn is associated with skin cancer and premature aging of the skin in adulthood. Cataracts in later life may also be secondary to too much sun. Most of the damage is caused by ultraviolet waves A and B (UVA and UVB). Unfortunately, sunburn is usually noticed too late, often a number of hours after exposure, when redness and pain develop. Given the risks, it makes sense to keep your baby away from excessive sunlight exposure and use sunscreen for children over the age of 6 months.

Hats with brims, long sleeves, and pants provide some sun protection. Bathing suits with long sleeves and pants, made of fabrics with higher sun protection factors than regular clothing, are very practical.

If your baby will tolerate wearing sunglasses, they will protect his eyes from the harmful rays of the sun. Make sure the label states that the sunglasses are 100% UV protective.

KEY POINT

Avoid prolonged sun exposure during the hours when the sun is the strongest: 10 a.m. to 2 p.m.

Sunscreens

Many sunscreens are available and approved for use in babies over 6 months. Sunscreens have simply not been tested on younger infants, so they have not received approval for the very young. No sunscreen is 100% protective, and all sunscreens should be applied frequently and liberally.

Most dermatologists recommend sunscreens with a sun protection factor (SPF) of at least 30. The SPF indicates how long a person can be exposed to sun before the skin burns. The higher the number, the longer the effect lasts. Protection varies depending on individual skin color and age — lighter skin is more susceptible to damage, and babies are likely to burn in less than the 20 to 30 minutes it takes for older individuals.

Sunscreen should be applied liberally at least 30 minutes before you go outside and reapplied every 2 to 3 hours, especially if your baby is in the water or perspiring a lot.

Insect Repellents

Mosquito bites are itchy and annoying — what's more, they occasionally become infected. The most effective way to avoid mosquito bites is to remain indoors, especially around dusk and dawn. However, when that is not a practical option, mosquito repellents and protective clothing should be worn. Some natural repellents, such as citronella, are available, but studies have shown that these do not provide adequate protection against mosquito bites. DEET is the most effective chemical mosquito repellent. The American Academy of Pediatrics (AAP) says DEET is safe, even in small children, when used as directed. According to the AAP, it can be used on babies older than 2 months in up to 30% concentration.

As with sunscreen, the number on the bottle indicates the duration of effectiveness: 10% DEET provides about 2 hours of protection; 30% provides about 5 hours of protection. Use the lowest percentage that will provide protection for the time your baby may be exposed.

DEET should be applied to all exposed areas, but the eyes, mouth, and open wounds should be avoided. Don't put DEET on the hands of little children, who are likely to put their fingers into their mouths and touch their eyes. DEET can also be applied to clothing. After coming back indoors, wash the DEET off your child's skin.

Remember that DEET and other mosquito repellents are not effective against some of the other insects we frequently encounter in the summer months, including bees, wasps, hornets, and ants.

DID YOU KNOW?

COMBINATION PRODUCTS

Avoid products that combine sunscreen and mosquito repellent. Sunscreen should be applied often and generously, while mosquito repellent should be used infrequently and sparingly.

DID YOU KNOW?

STANDING WATER

Remove potential breeding grounds for mosquitoes by getting rid of all standing water, for example, in outside toys, pails, and baskets.

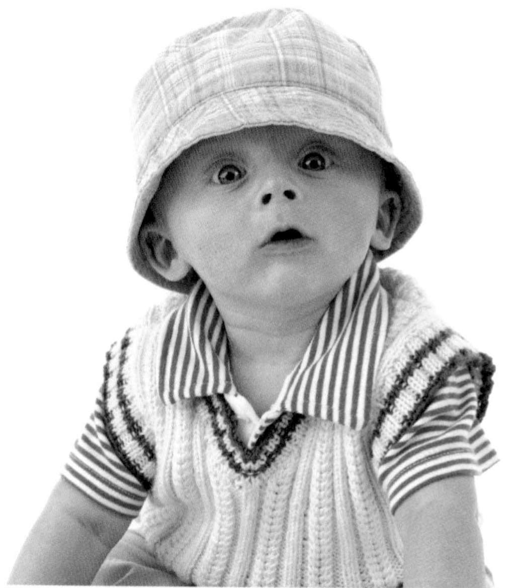

Returning to Work

Parenting is work! All mothers and fathers know that taking care of an infant is pretty much a full-time job. What "returning to work" really means is going back to paid employment outside of the home — adding to your already busy schedule.

Back in the workplace, you will be frequently torn between your home and work responsibilities. Leaving your baby for several hours a day can be very difficult emotionally and, sometimes, physically. But parents who stay at home full-time sometimes feel frustrated and underappreciated.

Making a Decision

Your decision to return to your previous job or start a new job rests on the specifics of your situation: your career goals, your sense of job satisfaction, financial pressures, and available options for child care. Make a decision that works best for your family, and realize that there is no perfect solution.

Advance Planning

To minimize stress and make the transition back to the workplace easier, advance planning is essential. Is the baby ready? Are you? Are all the supports you need in place?

Feeding

If your baby is still breast-feeding, you need to make sure he will drink expressed breast milk or formula from a bottle or cup while you are away. Many women take breast pumps to work and store expressed milk. Alternatively, slowly weaning the baby, partially or fully, from breast milk may facilitate your return to the workplace. Abrupt weaning can be very uncomfortable, so seek advice from your health-care provider or lactation consultant if it becomes necessary.

Employer Empathy

Understanding and empathetic employers and co-workers are highly desirable but not always easy to find. You may want to meet with your employer before you go back to work to discuss potential problems and solutions. For example, your work hours may now need to be more flexible. You will also need to work out a contingency plan for days when your child is ill and needs your direct care. Then there are

DID YOU KNOW?

PATERNITY LEAVE

Paternity leave is a wonderful option for some families. Some couples can stagger their hours so that one parent is always home with the baby.

the routine medical and dental appointments during the workday. Others in your workplace are likely also parents and aware of the issues of working parenthood.

Child Care

There are many reputable agencies to help families select and screen child-care workers. Obviously, they charge for their services. Your friends and acquaintances, especially those who have young children of their own, can be helpful resources, as can your health-care provider.

Regardless of the choice you make for child care, separation is often difficult. Innate factors, such as your baby's age and temperament, and external factors, such as familiarity with caregivers, will affect how your child adjusts. In general, despite a few tears from Mom, Dad, and baby, most families settle into the new routine quite easily.

In-Home Caregivers

By hiring a nanny or babysitter to come to your house, you allow your child to remain in familiar surroundings and may give yourself more flexibility in your work hours. Plus, you won't need to get the baby dressed, fed, and out the door while you are rushing to get ready for work.

However, some families feel that their personal space is invaded by having a "stranger" in their home. And an in-home nanny is usually a more expensive option than daycare, though it becomes more cost-effective if you have more than one young child at home. Bear in mind that if your nanny needs time off, you will have to make alternative arrangements, sometimes at very short notice. However, if your baby is sick, the nanny will be a constant and comforting caregiver.

Daycare Centers

In a regulated group daycare center, your baby will be cared for by trained professional child-care workers and exposed to other children, which provides opportunities for physical and social development. Daycare should provide a stimulating and enjoyable environment.

Most jurisdictions have stringent laws to regulate the size of daycare centers (the caregiver-to-child ratio), to establish safe facilities, and to ensure that staff members are adequately trained. There are also specific requirements for hygiene and sanitation. Nevertheless, the major disadvantage of daycare is the increased number of infections to which children are exposed. It is well documented that children in daycare contract more diseases than those who stay home. Most are common, minor viral illnesses, particularly gastroenteritis and colds. Daycare centers are usually very strict about excluding children who are ill with potentially infectious diseases, so if your child does become sick, you will have to make arrangements for an alternative caregiver to stay at home until he is no longer considered contagious.

KEY POINT

When seeking out a daycare center, look for an environment in which you think your baby will thrive. Talk to parents who have children in the daycare, as well as to the caregivers who work there.

Home Daycare Centers

Home daycare centers are child-care programs run out of people's houses. They often have more flexible hours, and they usually take just a few children of varying ages, thus providing a smaller and more intimate environment. Because there are fewer children, the risk of infection is lower. In many jurisdictions, home daycare centers are registered with government agencies and evaluated by the appropriate authorities on a regular basis.

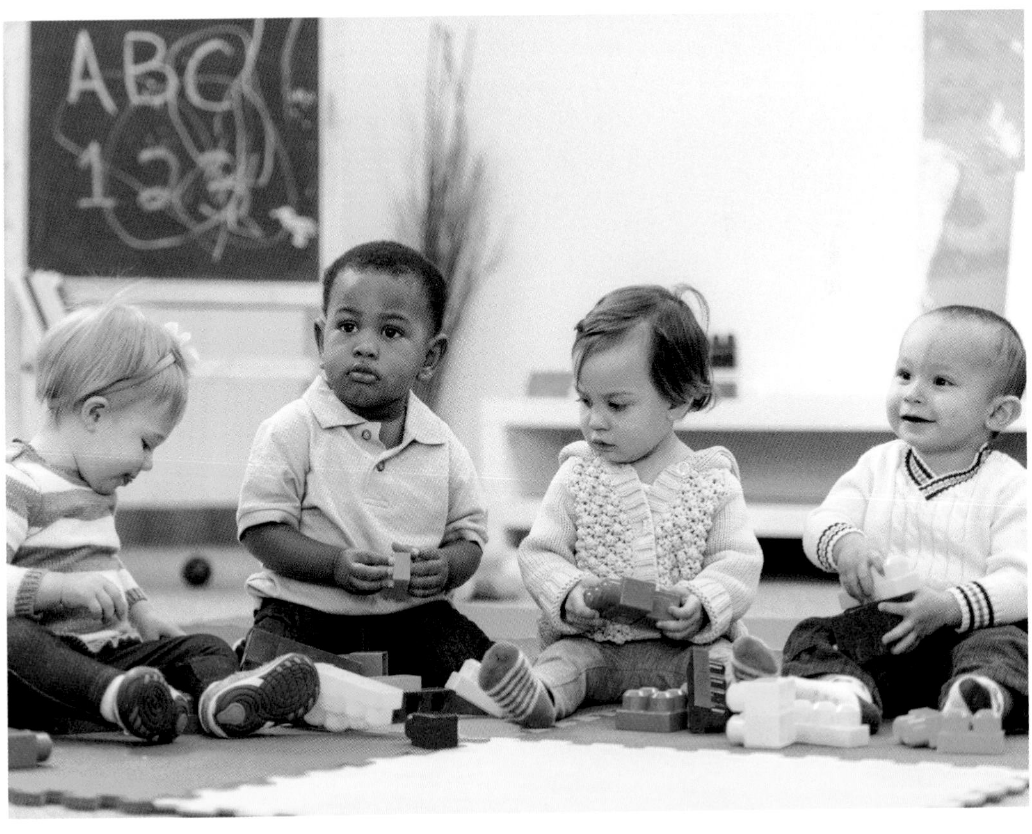

Frequently Asked Questions

Every time I leave my baby, he gets upset. How am I ever going to return to work?

It's normal for a baby to miss his mother at this age. It's also normal for mothers to be upset. After all, strong bonds have been formed between you. Only you know whether returning to work is your best option. But if it is, the transition is unlikely to be perfectly smooth — it will be an adjustment for both of you. Take comfort knowing that, in the end, both mother and baby do adjust. The best way to handle returning to work is to ensure that your baby's caregivers are both capable and affectionate.

My 10-month-old daughter has already caught two colds since starting daycare. Is that normal?

For the first few months of life, babies are protected from most childhood infections by antibodies obtained from their mothers before birth. But these antibodies don't last forever. In the second 6 months, babies become susceptible to common childhood infections. At daycare centers, there is ample opportunity to be exposed to them. Getting colds is a part of growing up. Immunity from common childhood illnesses is acquired by infection with the viruses that cause them.

As my baby approaches his first birthday, he looks thinner than before. Is there something wrong?

Probably not. Children tend to lose their baby fat at this age. They are more mobile and therefore burn more calories. You should be concerned only if your baby is actually losing weight or has persisting symptoms such as prolonged cough or diarrhea.

When and how do I start to bathe my baby in a regular bathtub?

Babies are pretty slippery when wet. While it won't harm her to slip underwater momentarily, neither of you is likely to enjoy the experience much. It's best to wait until she can sit properly on her own before switching to a full-size bathtub; otherwise, you won't have enough hands for the job. Make sure the water is the right temperature: comfortably warm to your hand but neither hot nor chilly. Bathing should be fun: a few floating bath toys will convert the bath into a delightful playground. Be prepared. Have everything you need — towels, washcloths, baby shampoo — ready to go. Finally, there must always be a lifeguard on duty. Never leave a baby unattended in the bathtub, even for a moment.

My baby's first tooth didn't erupt until he was 8 months old. Now his teeth seem crooked. What's wrong?

Nothing. Of all a baby's milestones, the eruption of the teeth is the most variable. The lower incisors usually appear first, but many healthy babies get their upper incisors first. In the beginning, baby teeth often appear crooked. But, as the full set appears, the teeth act as splints for one another, straightening them nicely. By the time they attend nursery school or preschool, children will have their full set of 20 primary teeth.

My daughter lost her baby hair, and it has not grown back. Should I be concerned?

Many babies lose some or all of their hair during the first few months. The hair that grows back may be quite different, both in color and texture, than the hair they were born with. Some babies remain bald for many months, sometimes well into the second year of life. This is most common in very fair babies. Rest assured that your baby's hair will come in eventually, and that infantile baldness does not predict hair loss in adulthood.

Now that my baby can cruise the furniture, I've noticed that he appears flat-footed. How could he have developed fallen arches so soon?

Flat feet are normal during infancy. The muscles and ligaments that will later maintain the foot's arch are too loose and flexible to do so at this age. They can't prevent the flattening of the foot when it is bearing weight. Over the course of several years, the joints in the foot gradually tighten, and the arch is then maintained.

When my sister visits, she usually brings along her own young toddler. My 11-month-old daughter notices him, but doesn't seem interested in playing. Is my daughter antisocial, or even autistic?

Most children don't engage in interactive play until they are beyond infancy. Most 11-month-old babies will notice and react to other children, but their play is "parallel" rather than interactive. On the other hand, it is reasonable to expect your daughter to notice her cousin, make eye contact, and play games such as peekaboo with adults.

I hear that obesity is a major problem in children. Should I be limiting my 10-month-old to low-fat dairy products? Is there anything else I can do to prevent him from being obese when he grows up?

You are correct: the prevalence of childhood obesity is rapidly rising. Obese children often become obese adults, with multiple serious medical complications, so this is a serious issue. However, the first two years of life are a time of extremely rapid growth, and your child's weight will triple in the first year alone! For optimal growth and development, your baby's food intake should not be limited, nor should fat, an important building block, be restricted in any way.

CHAPTER 9

Protecting Your Baby

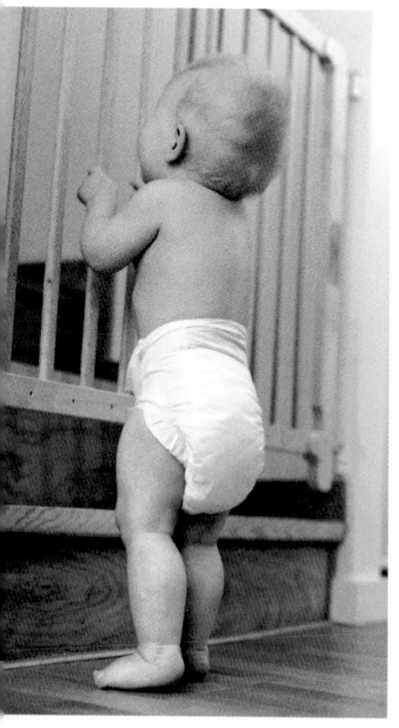

One of a parent's worst nightmares is that their child will injure herself, and for good reason: injuries are the greatest cause of death and disability for children in North America. Children generally acquire motor skills long before they have the intellectual ability to recognize danger. For this reason, it is very important to make sure that your child's environment is rendered as safe as possible. Common sense, in the form of appropriate supervision, advance planning, and "childproofing" your home, will prevent most accidents. When accidents do occur, you can be prepared to help your child by learning first aid.

Childproofing Basics

Even the most obsessive parent will not be able to supervise every second of a baby's first year. Bearing this in mind, the three most important factors influencing accidents are your baby's age, temperament, and environment. Because you have little control over the first two factors, most of your efforts should be geared toward removing hazards from your baby's surroundings.

DID YOU KNOW?

COMMON ACCIDENTS

Suffocation and choking are the injuries that most often result in death in the first year of life. Falling is the one that most frequently results in hospitalization. Other common accidents include burns, drowning, and poisoning. Many of these injuries occur in the home.

- **See like a child:** To minimize the risk of accidents, try to see the world through the eyes of an inquisitive baby. Get down on all fours and see what you could potentially pull down or grasp. You also need to anticipate the dangers that might accompany each new developmental milestone. For example, you won't want to remember that the first time your baby rolled over was when she fell from the changing table!
- **Look for hazards:** Pay attention to hazards that can injure your baby, such as sharp corners, cords for blinds or curtains, and electrical outlets and wires. Staircases can be extremely dangerous. Small objects, including toys with small pieces, small batteries, jewelry, and stones, are potential choking hazards; make sure they are inaccessible.
- **Remove temptations:** When your baby starts to move around in the second 6 months, be aware that she is

not developmentally capable of remembering that you told her not to play with the electrical cord, even if you have told her 20 times. She is not being "naughty"; she is merely behaving like any other inquisitive 9-month-old.
- **Supervise:** Certainly childproof your baby's environment as meticulously as possible, but there is no substitute for vigilance and supervision. Studies suggest that babies are most at risk when you are distracted. Unless they are asleep in their cribs, infants should not be left alone. Babies should never be left alone in the bathtub or near water — not even for a second. Children can drown in only an inch (2.5 cm) of water. Nor should babies be left unsupervised with young children, who are notorious for poking and prodding or trying to feed the baby inappropriate food as soon as the adult leaves the room.

DID YOU KNOW?

NO HOT DRINKS

Never drink or hold hot liquid when holding your child — a spill could scald her. It can be helpful to use a cup with a lid.

Making Your Home Safe for Your Baby

Here are some guidelines for making your home safe for your baby, room by room.

Bedroom

Safe Cribs and Bedding

When buying a crib, whether new or used, make sure it meets current safety standards. Cribs made before 2011 were often made with drop-down side rails, which are no longer considered safe because there is an associated risk of entrapment, suffocation, or strangulation.

A mattress should be firm and should fit snugly into the crib, with no room for tiny limbs to get stuck — generally no more than two finger widths between the mattress and the crib wall. Set the mattress lower when your baby starts to sit up and at its lowest position when she starts to pull to a standing position.

When you put your baby down to sleep, she will need a fitted crib sheet, but no pillows, bumper pads, comforters, stuffed toys, or soft objects, all of which have been shown to increase the risk of sudden infant death syndrome (SIDS).

Cribs should be placed away from the window, clear of blind or curtain cords, which can strangle an older baby. If you use a crib mobile, ensure that your baby cannot reach it.

DID YOU KNOW?

SIDS PREVENTION

Most parents want to decorate the crib with baby gifts, but when it is time for sleep, take all the pretty things out. To minimize the risk of sudden infant death syndrome (SIDS), put your baby to sleep on her back, lightly clothed, with only a sheet for bedding. Do not overheat her. The risks increase if you bed-share with your baby, especially if you or your partner smokes, is significantly overweight, or has consumed alcohol, drugs, or any medications that would make you drowsy.

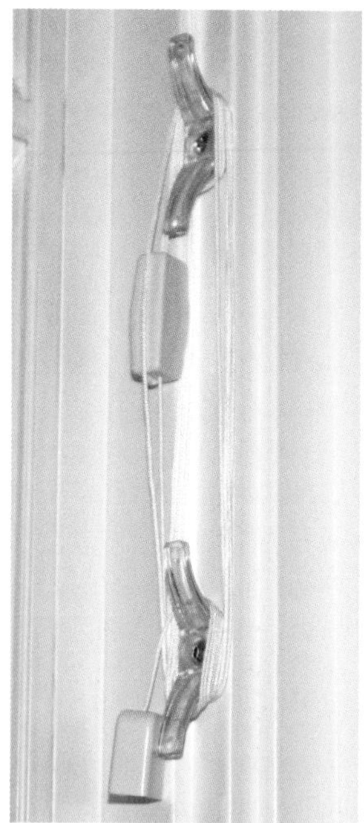

All curtain and blind cords should be clamped to the window frame, far out of your child's reach.

Diaper Changing Tables

Never leave your baby unattended on a changing table or bed — you never know when she will decide to roll for the first time. Keep diapers and a fresh set of clothing within easy reach, and always keep one hand on the baby.

Toy Boxes

Injuries are occasionally caused when a toy box lid falls on a child's head, body, or little fingers, and children can get stuck inside. The safest ones have no lid. Better yet, store your child's toys in open and easily accessible places.

Bathroom

Bathtub

Never, ever leave your infant or toddler unsupervised in the bath. Children can drown in as little as 1 inch (2.5 cm) of water. If you have to answer the telephone or doorbell, wrap your child in a towel and take her with you.

Non-Slip Mats and Spout Covers

Use a non-slip mat on the bottom of the bathtub. Protective covers for the spout are also available.

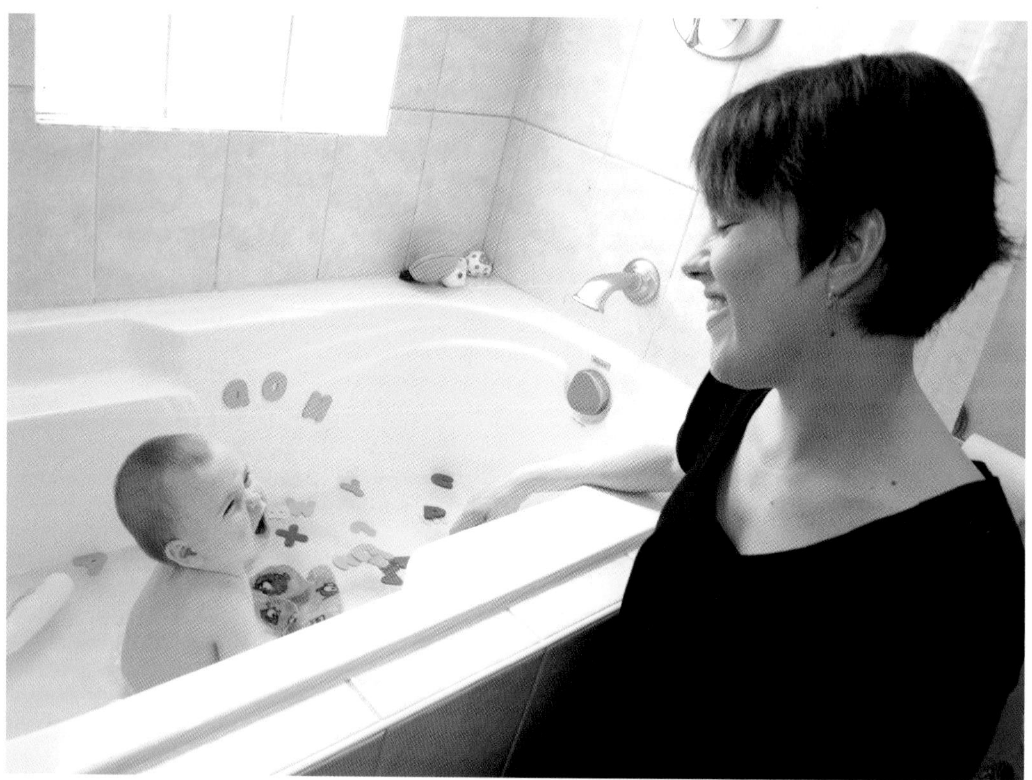

Toilet Lids

Infants and young toddlers are fascinated by the toilet — that is, until you want them to use it during toilet training! To prevent your child from playing in the toilet or even falling in, purchase a latching mechanism to keep the lid closed.

Medicine Cabinet

Make sure your medicine cabinet is out of reach and has a child-resistant lock to keep inquisitive fingers out. Even though all medications should have a safety cap, they still need to be locked away. Do not leave any type of medication, even vitamins, outside of the locked cabinet, and especially not in purses or bags. Don't refer to your child's medication as candy — they may seek it out. Soaps, shampoos, perfumes, and deodorants should also be kept out of reach.

Kitchen

Stoves and Ovens

Pots on the stove should be on the rear plates, with the handles pointing inward — pulling up on the handle of a pot or pan can result in a tragic scald burn. The oven door should be well insulated (the same is true for the glass fronts of fireplaces) and should never be left open.

Microwave Ovens

It is best not to use microwave ovens to warm up your baby's bottle; the heat is not evenly distributed, and some parts of the milk may burn your baby's mouth. If you do use one to heat up food, mix it thoroughly and test it before offering it.

Cupboard Locks

All dangerous objects, including kitchen cleaners and sharp utensils, should be kept in a cabinet out of reach and protected with a child-resistant lock; in fact, it's a good idea to put child-resistant locks on all of your kitchen cabinets. Place dangerous items in the upper cabinets and safe items in the lower, more reachable cabinets.

DID YOU KNOW?

WATER TEMPERATURE

Water heaters in North American homes are often set to 140°F (60°C). At this temperature, severe burns can occur within 1 to 5 seconds of contact with water! To prevent scalding burns, set your home water heater to no more than 120°F (50°C). At temperatures below 120°F (50°C), water will take 2 to 10 minutes to cause a severe burn, which gives you much more time to prevent scalding by getting your baby out of the water.

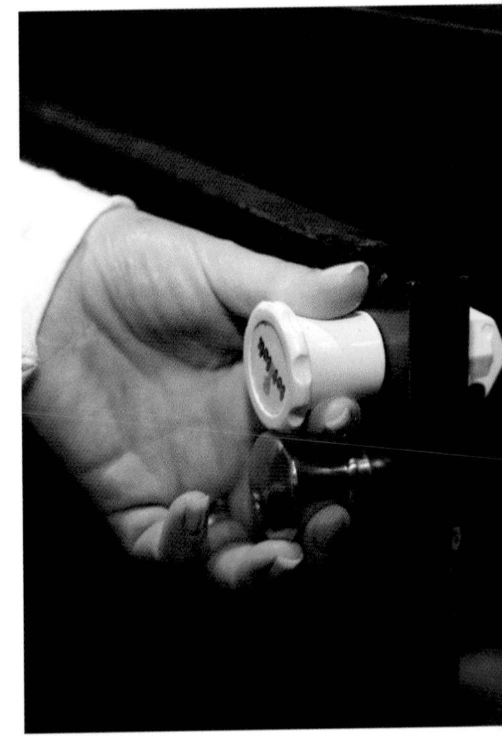

DID YOU KNOW?

TOYS IN THE KITCHEN

Keep a large container of toys in the kitchen to distract your baby while you're cooking, and create a "safe" zone — for example, a playpen, high chair, or exersaucer. Small refrigerator magnet toys are a potential choking hazard, so avoid them.

Table Mats

Use table mats or placemats instead of tablecloths, which can be pulled down with all of their contents landing on top of your child.

Laundry Room

The laundry room should be off limits; nevertheless, ensure that the washer and dryer doors are always closed and that all detergents and bleach are kept in secured cupboards, well out of reach. Laundry detergent and dishwashing "pods" are often brightly colored and resemble candy. They are potentially toxic when held in sweaty little hands or placed in mouths. Ensure that they are stored well out of reach in a locked cupboard. Switch off and put away the iron when you are done with it.

Further Precautions

There are many other steps you can take to make your home as safe as possible.

- **Electrical sockets:** Plastic covers inserted in all unused electrical sockets will prevent your baby from sticking her fingers or other objects into them. Appliances not in use should be unplugged, and any electrical cords kept far out of reach.
- **Heat sources:** Avoid using space heaters if possible and keep all heaters out of reach of children. Matches and lighters should be locked away. Installing a fire extinguisher in the home is highly recommended.
- **Smoke and carbon monoxide detectors:** Smoke and carbon monoxide detectors should be installed on every level of the home, at a minimum. They need to be carefully maintained and regularly checked.
- **Furniture:** Sharp edges on furniture are particularly dangerous when your baby starts to crawl and cruise around. Coffee tables are notorious for this problem. Edges can be covered with protectors. (Or remove the offending furniture altogether!)
- **Appliances and bookcases:** Heavy appliances such as televisions should be carefully secured and preferably placed out of reach. Bookcases and dressers can be screwed into the wall so they don't topple over onto the child.

- **Window hardware:** Windows should have safety catches and screens attached. All blind and curtain cords should be carefully wrapped or clipped out of reach to prevent strangulation.
- **Doors and screens:** Be sure to keep all doors and screens secured with child-resistant locks. Glass doors should be marked with decals to prevent your child from walking into them.
- **Trash cans and plastic bags:** Trash containers need childproof lids. Never leave plastic bags lying around: your child might place one over her head, causing suffocation.
- **Weapons:** Do not keep weapons in the home. If you must, ensure that firearms are not loaded and are carefully locked up.

DID YOU KNOW?

STAIRS

Stairs are particularly hazardous for infants and toddlers. Place gates at both the top and the bottom before your baby starts crawling. Make sure your gates meet current safety standards and are properly secured. The gate at the top must be secured to the wall so that it will not give way if pushed.

Safety-Proofing Baby Equipment

Precautions also apply to baby equipment — playpens, jumpers, exersaucers, and toys.

Playpens

Playpens should always be opened completely so they don't collapse later with the baby inside. The mattress should fit the base snugly. The openings in the mesh sides should be too small for your baby to get anything caught in them. Make sure your baby cannot climb out of the playpen.

KEY POINT

Do not use baby walkers. They have been banned in many jurisdictions because they have caused numerous injuries and some deaths from falls down stairs.

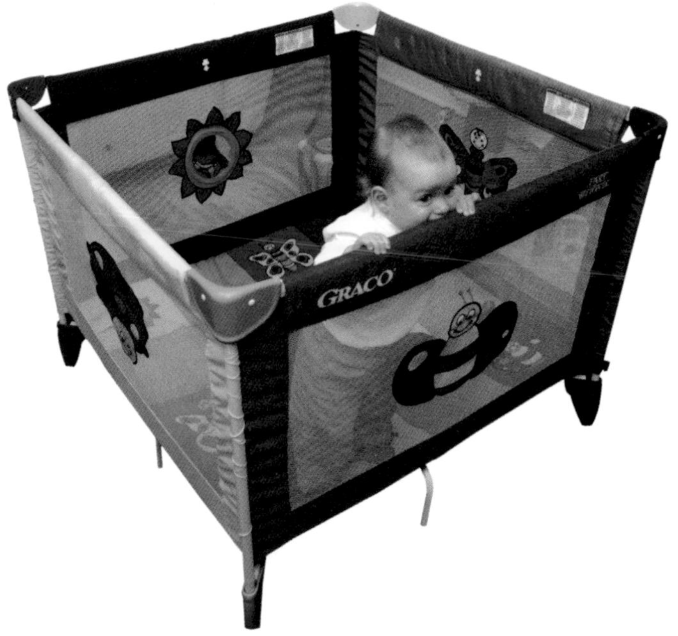

DID YOU KNOW?

PETS

Children are more commonly bitten by pets than adults are. The arrival of a new baby is a time for extreme caution, even with a trusted, gentle canine or feline family member. Do not leave your child alone with your pet until much later. Bites can occur during play. When your baby becomes mobile, keep her away from the cat's litter box, as the litter is a possible source of infection and a potential choking hazard.

KEY POINT

Knowing how to respond in an emergency can save a life. The techniques you are taught will allow you to remain calm and provide appropriate first aid to your child while help is on its way.

Jumpers and Exersaucers

Be careful to fasten jumpers securely in such a way that your baby cannot bump up against anything. Exersaucers should be placed far away from any dangers, such as window cords and stairs.

Toys

Toys need to be age-appropriate — check the packaging. No toy small enough to fit in your baby's mouth is safe! Check from time to time to make sure the eyes and nose on your child's soft toys are still firmly attached. Latex balloons are dangerous; if one pops, the plastic can be inhaled, suffocating the child.

Tiny objects act as magnets for little hands and can cause your baby to choke if she swallows one. This is a particular danger in homes with older children, who tend to leave small toys lying around. Teach older siblings to pick up all the pieces of their toys. If they can't clean up all by themselves, make sure to help them. When a toy involves small pieces, it's better if your older child plays with it on the kitchen table or anywhere above your baby's reach.

Learning First Aid

Despite your most conscientious efforts to childproof your home and supervise your baby, injuries can occur at any time. Having a prepared plan of action for an emergency will certainly beat making decisions when you're upset and panicking. Keep a list of emergency telephone numbers, including your local poison control center and family physician's office, clearly posted in a couple of places.

Basic Life Support

We strongly advise new parents to take a basic life support (BLS) course that deals with infants (less than 1 year) and young children (1 to 8 years of age). Try to take this course before your baby arrives — it will be tough to find time afterwards. Reading about it is not a good substitute. You need to practice on mannequins until you feel confident that you can perform the necessary techniques.

Choking

Choking is the most common accidental cause of death in infancy. Solid objects, such as toys or coins, are not the only cause of choking. If milk or food goes down "the wrong way" into the windpipe and lungs rather than into the esophagus and stomach, it can lead to choking. Usually, this will be followed by a coughing spell with some gagging. Parents must be prepared to help children who are choking — a skill that can be learned in a BLS course.

HOW TO: Prevent Choking

As always, prevention is the best treatment. To minimize the risk of a serious choking episode, take these precautions:

- Grate, blend, mash, or chop your child's food into very small pieces (less than ½ inch/1 cm).
- Slice round, firm foods, such as hot dog slices or grapes, lengthwise into quarters.
- Remove small objects and pieces of toys from the baby's surroundings. Pieces of broken balloon, button-type batteries, and coins are likely to cause major problems. Keep your purse or wallet out of reach.
- Remove toys marked "Not for children under 3 years" – they are usually a choking hazard.

Burns

There are many ways in which a baby can accidentally get burned: pulling a pan of hot liquid down on herself, touching a glass fireplace protector, a heater, or an oven door, or getting caught in a house fire. Once again, these serious injuries can be prevented with some straightforward childproofing techniques.

Treating Burns

- If it is anything more serious than a mild first-degree burn (for example, if the skin blisters), bring your baby to the emergency department.
- Cool the area as soon as possible — the skin will continue burning until it is cooled down. Cold water (but not ice water) is easiest to use. Either dip an extremity into a bowl of cold water for at least 10 to 20 minutes or wrap a cool wet cloth around the burnt area.
- Remove any constricting clothing before the swelling starts, but if clothing is stuck to the burnt area, do not pull it off.

KEY POINT

Do not use ice on burns — it can cause further damage to the tissues. And don't apply butter, creams, grease, or powder — these can make the burn worse, despite what our grandmothers told us.

- Cover the burn with sterile gauze (if you have it in your first aid kit) or a clean sheet or towel.
- Give the child acetaminophen or ibuprofen for pain relief.

Cuts and Bleeding

Bleeding from cuts and other injuries is uncommon in the first year but becomes more common as your baby becomes more mobile and adventurous. Cuts on the forehead and chin are not uncommon and can bleed quite a bit!

KEY POINT

All wounds caused by a bite (animal or human) that breaks the skin should be seen by a doctor.

Treating Cuts and Bleeding

- Cover the wound with a clean cloth and apply pressure for a few minutes to stop any active bleeding.
- Rinse the wound with water, washing out any gravel or dirt.
- If bleeding is ongoing, cover the wound with a clean cloth and apply firm pressure while elevating the area above the level of the heart. If the wound is on an extremity, lay the baby down and hold the extremity up. If it is on the head or face, sit the baby upright. If the area of the wound cannot be raised above the level of the heart, simply continue to apply pressure.
- If the wound is very dirty, with foreign material embedded, it may need to be carefully cleaned. If the wound is gaping, or bleeding continues, stitches may be required. Seek medical attention immediately.

KEY POINT

Keep all medicines and other potential poisons in their original containers. Take your medicine out of sight of your infant, and discard any leftover prescription medications at your local pharmacy. Be particularly vigilant when away from home, at the grandparents' house, for example.

Poisoning

Many poisonous substances can be found in kitchens, bathrooms, and laundry rooms. Poisons can be swallowed, breathed in, or absorbed through the skin. Keep the telephone number of your local poison control center readily available.

Treating Poisoning

- If your child can't be roused and isn't breathing, begin CPR and call 911 immediately.
- If your child cannot be roused but is breathing normally, place her on her side to ensure that she doesn't choke if she vomits.
- Look for a source of poison in the near vicinity (for example, a medication container or a chewed houseplant), then call the poison control center and

tell them the names of any substances that may have been ingested or inhaled.

- If anything is still in your baby's mouth, remove it immediately, but don't throw it away — it may help identify the poison.
- If you suspect that your baby has swallowed a chemical poison, wash her lips with water. Do not give her more than a few sips of water before getting advice from the poison control center or your health-care provider.
- If you think your baby has spilled a chemical on her skin, remove her clothes and rinse the skin with lukewarm water for at least 10 minutes.
- If you think she may have inhaled poisonous fumes, move her out into the fresh air.
- If a poisonous substance has splashed in her eye, rinse the eye with lukewarm water for as long as you can (up to 15 minutes).
- If your child vomits, try to keep a sample to take with you to the hospital. Do not give your child anything to make her vomit. If she has ingested a caustic substance (contained in many detergents and kitchen cleaners), inducing vomiting may cause more damage.

KEY POINT

Syrup of ipecac is no longer recommended to induce vomiting under any circumstances — if you have any at home, get rid of it.

GUIDE TO: Household Poison Hazards

Keep these products locked in a high cupboard, out of sight and out of reach:

- All medicines, especially iron supplements, vitamins, aspirin, and acetaminophen
- Cleaning products, including drain cleaner, furniture polish, dishwashing soap, laundry "pods," and bleach
- Pesticides and herbicides, such as weed killer, ant traps, and mouse and rat poison
- Motor vehicle products, such as gasoline, antifreeze, and windshield wiper fluid
- Paint, paint thinners, glue, kerosene, and other solvents and fuels
- Mothballs

Frequently Asked Questions

Are infant bath seats and rings safe?

In the United States, there have been more than 100 deaths and many more reported near-miss drownings over the last 20 years related to the use of infant bath seats or rings. Accidents typically occur when the seat becomes unstable and tips over or the baby slips through or climbs out while the caregiver has briefly left her unattended or in the care of a sibling. For this reason, many authorities, including Health Canada, discourage their use. The U.S. Consumer Product Safety Commission recommends that infant bath seats or rings should not be used unless they were manufactured after December 2010 and meet current safety standards. It is essential that you maintain close, constant supervision for the entire time your baby remains in the bath.

We have a 6-month-old son and would like to get a dog. Do you have any suggestions?

For millions of families, life is richly enhanced by the presence of a family pet. By all means, get one — just not necessarily now. Remember that puppies are babies too. Training and caring for them takes a lot of work. With a 6-month-old in the home, you are probably stretched pretty thin already. So first make sure you are really ready for a dog.

If, after careful reflection, you still want a dog now, pick a breed known for its good disposition and tolerance of children. Socialize your dog with people, especially other children, and with other dogs. A well-behaved dog will be a lot easier to deal with, so enroll in a puppy obedience program. Never leave your baby and the dog alone together. Be sure that the dog's food is out of your baby's reach: turf wars can get ugly, and your baby may not appreciate the fact that tasting the dog's dinner isn't very smart. Finally, dog feces must be cleaned up immediately.

My 10-month-old daughter was crawling on our deck and got a large sliver in her hand. What is the best way to remove it?

First, gather everything you are likely to need: gauze pads (or cotton balls), a sewing needle, tweezers, antibiotic ointment, and a Band-Aid. Because babies don't appreciate the advantages of sliver removal, an assistant, if available, will be a good idea.

Cleanse the area with soap and water. Using the needle, further expose the protruding end of the sliver as best as you can. Grab that end with the tweezers and pull out the sliver. Afterwards, liberally apply antibiotic ointment and cover the sore with a Band-Aid.

If the sliver appears to have lodged very deep and is unlikely to be easily removed, consult a health-care provider.

If your baby has multiple tiny (1⁄32 to 1⁄16 inch/1 to 2 mm) slivers that are very superficial, it might be best to leave them alone, although you can still apply antibiotic ointment. The potential tissue damage caused by the attempt to remove the slivers may cause your baby greater distress than the slivers themselves. They will grow out in time.

CHAPTER 10

Caring for Your Sick Baby

Caring for a sick child is, without a doubt, one of the most distressing parts of being a parent. While you can treat some illnesses at home, others need to be addressed by health-care providers in their medical offices, clinics, or emergency departments.

KEY POINT

Emergency situations, of course, require immediate care in a hospital; be especially alert for "red flag" signs and symptoms.

▷ Red Flag Signs and Symptoms

If your baby shows these red flag signs and symptoms, seek immediate medical attention:

- Your young infant (3 months or younger) has a fever.
- Your baby is refusing to feed and/or vomiting, with decreased urination and dry eyes, dry tongue, and lack of tears (suggestive of dehydration).
- He is lethargic, with a decreased level of consciousness.
- He is uncharacteristically irritable or inconsolable.
- He is breathing rapidly or finding it difficult to breathe, suggested by flaring of the nostrils or "in-drawing" of the skin between the ribs or below the ribcage with each breath.
- His limbs are jerking abnormally, especially if the jerking does not stop when the limb is held (suggestive of a convulsion or seizure).

Fever

At some time, every child will experience fever. Fever is the most common reason for a child to be brought for emergency care. While most fevers are the result of a self-limited and benign illness, almost all parents will at some point worry that a more serious disease is causing their baby's fever. Your anxiety will be reduced if you understand how fevers develop and know how to take your child's temperature.

"Normal" Temperature

Technically defined, a fever is an elevation in body temperature; however, "normal" body temperature varies

What Is a Fever?

ROUTE MEASURED	TEMPERATURE
Rectal	> 100.4°F (38.0°C)
Axillary (under arm)	> 99°F (37.2°C)
Oral (under tongue)	> 99.5°F (37.5°C)
Tympanic (ear)	> 99.5°F (37.5°C)

according to where it is measured and when it is measured, as well as by the surrounding environment and your child's clothing.

When to Be Concerned

Fever itself does not cause brain damage or any other significant problems, as some people believe. Nor does the height of a fever necessarily indicate the severity of illness. In fact, some serious infections may be accompanied by a minimally elevated or even lower-than-normal body temperature.

More important than the height of the fever is your baby's behavior. While most feverish babies are cranky and clingy, with decreased appetite, be especially concerned if your baby does not show interest in or awareness of his surroundings, does not make appropriate eye contact, or is inconsolable. Contact a health-care provider immediately if these behaviors accompany a fever.

DID YOU KNOW?

FEBRILE SEIZURES

While many parents are concerned about the potentially harmful effects of an elevated body temperature, they are especially frightened by fever-induced convulsions. Called febrile seizures, these convulsions are relatively common — about one in 20 children between 6 months and 5 years of age will have one. These events, while scary, almost always have minimal consequences for the child.

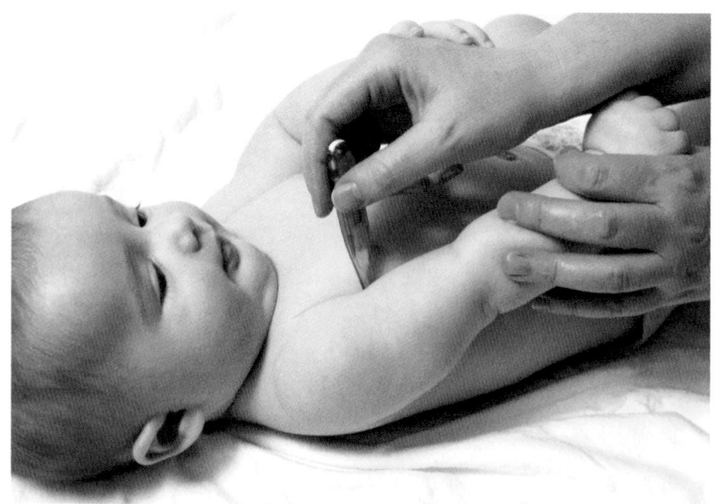

GUIDE TO: Taking Your Baby's Temperature

The type of thermometer and the route you should use to measure a child's temperature depend on his age, the circumstances, and the equipment available:

Type of Thermometer

- **Mercury:** Mercury thermometers are not recommended because of the potential for mercury exposure if the thermometer breaks. In addition, they have to remain in place longer before they record the correct temperature.
- **Digital:** Digital thermometers are safe, easy to use, and inexpensive. They are ready to read in less than a minute, which is helpful with a squirmy baby.
- **Tympanic (ear):** Tympanic thermometers are convenient, but are less reliable in children under 2 years of age. They give a reading in a few seconds, but are much more expensive than simple plastic digital thermometers.

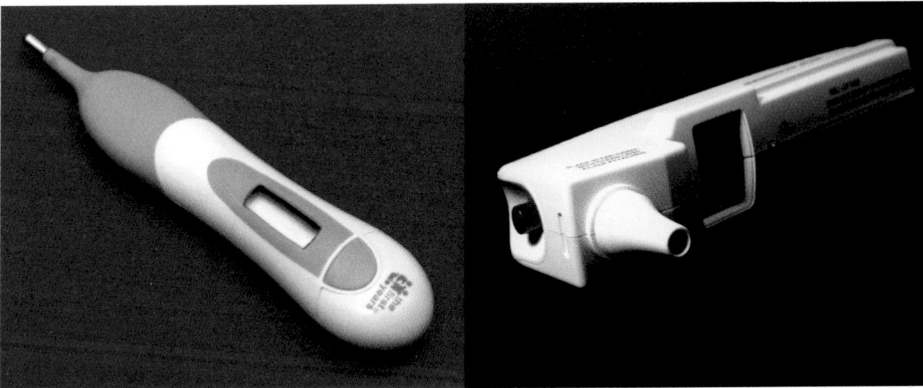

Route

- **Rectal:** Rectal temperature measurement is the most accurate method for young infants and is therefore the preferred route in the first 3 months. Place the baby on his back and lubricate the bulb of the thermometer with petroleum jelly. Lifting his legs up against his tummy, pinch the thermometer $\frac{1}{2}$ to $\frac{3}{4}$ inch (1 to 2 cm) from the tip of the bulb and gently insert it into the anus up to your pinched fingers. Parents are often nervous about this technique, but it is really very safe.
- **Axillary (under arm):** Axillary temperature measurement is convenient but is also the most unreliable. To take your child's temperature this way, place the tip of a digital oral or rectal thermometer in the armpit, and tuck the child's arm snugly against his chest.
- **Oral (under tongue):** By 4 to 5 years of age, children will usually cooperate with oral temperature measurement, which requires keeping the thermometer under the tongue.
- **Tympanic (ear):** Tympanic thermometers must fit easily inside the child's ear canal.

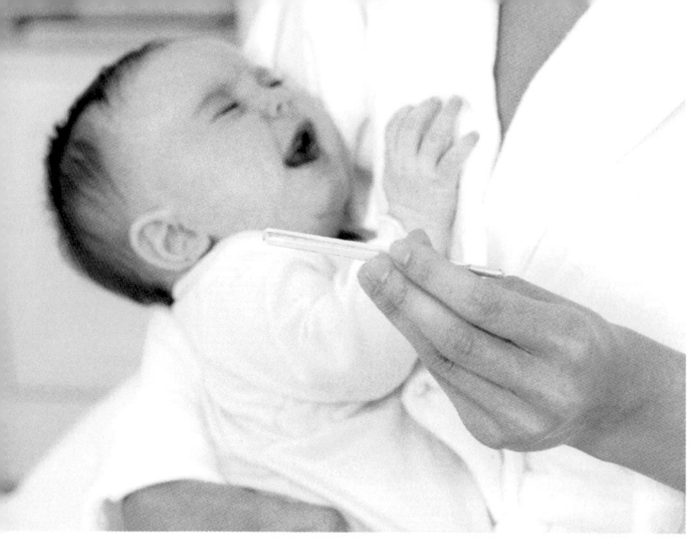

Fever in Young Infants

Fever in young infants, particularly those under 3 months of age, is cause for concern, in part because the child's immune system is immature and in part because the child has few ways to exhibit signs of serious illness. While more than 90% of feverish infants under 3 months of age have a self-resolving, uncomplicated viral infection, health-care providers will frequently perform a number of tests to look for potentially serious infections, such as meningitis, bloodstream infections, and urinary tract infections.

Reducing Risk

Your baby is at a slightly increased risk of infection in the first 2 to 3 months of life because his immune system is still developing. However, he has the benefit of much of your immunity because your antibodies crossed through the placenta into his bloodstream during fetal development. By giving him the recommended immunizations at the recommended times, you will help him to develop his own immunity to some rare but potentially devastating diseases.

KEY POINT

Aspirin (ASA) should not be given to children because of the risk of Reye's syndrome, a serious condition that can cause liver and brain injury.

Fever Red Flags

See a health-care provider immediately if your baby has these signs and symptoms in addition to a fever:

- He is less than 3 months of age.
- He does not interact appropriately.
- He is difficult to rouse, poorly responsive, or limp.
- He is inconsolable or appears to be in pain.
- He refuses to eat and drink.
- He is behaving as if his neck is stiff.
- He is having difficulty breathing.
- He has developed purple "spots" or bruises on his skin.

Also seek help if the fever has persisted for 2 to 3 days and your instincts tell you that your baby is "not himself."

Managing a Fever

Remember that most fevers in infants are caused by benign, self-limited viral infections that your baby can and will fight off by himself. Most fevers due to viral infections can be managed at home.

1. Determine if a fever is, in fact, present by taking your baby's temperature.
2. Comfort and cool your baby. Dress him lightly in a diaper and vest to allow body heat to escape.
3. Do not give your baby a cold water bath or sponge him with alcohol. The cold water is likely to be uncomfortable and can make him shiver; the alcohol can be absorbed into the body through the skin.
4. Offer your baby frequent feedings; fever causes increased loss of water.
5. Administer over-the-counter medications. The primary function of medication is to provide comfort for the child, not to eliminate the elevated body temperature. Acetaminophen (Tylenol, Tempra) and ibuprofen (Advil, Motrin) are safe and effective treatments for fever. There isn't much difference among these medications, which come in drops, syrups, suppositories, and chewable tablets for older children. The dosage for acetaminophen and ibuprofen is weight-based.

KEY POINT

Don't wait until 3 a.m. to work out what the appropriate dose is — calculate it ahead of time!

Common Cold

Healthy children may have 8 to 10 colds a year in the first years of life, and infants who have older siblings or are in daycare may seem to have a permanent cold. Colds are caused by a variety of viruses that are present throughout the year but are more common during the fall and winter months. Nasal congestion, clear to yellow/green nasal discharge, cough, fever, and mild sore throat are common symptoms.

Most colds last from a few days to a week or two and resolve on their own. For a typical common cold, an infant will not need to see his health-care provider.

Treating Colds

Acetaminophen (Tylenol, Tempra) or ibuprofen (Advil, Motrin) can be helpful to treat discomfort and fever. If your baby is less than 3 months old, have him assessed by a health-care provider before giving him any medication.

KEY POINT

Over-the-counter decongestants, cough suppressants, and antihistamines should not be used — they are ineffective in young children and have the potential for serious side effects. Antibiotics, which treat bacterial infections, have no role in treating a cold.

▷ Common Cold Red Flags

If your infant has any of the following complications from a cold, he should be seen by a health-care provider:

- He is breathing rapidly or with difficulty.
- He is listless and lacks interest in his surroundings.
- He has a persistent fever that has lasted more than 48 hours. (Infants under 3 months should see a doctor in any case of fever.)
- He cannot feed or keep fluids down.

Wheezing

Wheezing is a whistling or sighing noise made by air passing through narrowed small air passages in the lungs. Usually detected by a stethoscope, wheezing may sometimes be heard by the unaided ear. The sound of wheezing is quite different from the snoring noise heard when your baby breathes in with a congested nose from a cold.

One common reason for wheezing in infants is bronchiolitis, a viral infection that causes inflammation and narrowing of the small air passages in the lungs, leading to obstruction of airflow. Bronchiolitis is very common, especially in winter, and usually accompanies cold symptoms in adults or older children. But in young infants, who have smaller air passages, it often results in wheezing and difficulty breathing. Many infants will have cold symptoms before the wheezing begins, and they may have been in contact with someone with a cold.

Repeated episodes of wheezing in infancy are often a sign of asthma, which can develop in about 10% of young children. It is more common in babies whose families have a strong history of asthma, eczema, or hay fever. An asthma attack can be set off by a cold and can look almost identical to an episode of bronchiolitis. Once a child has had a couple of episodes of wheezing, especially if he responds well to puffers, he is usually considered to have asthma.

Both bronchiolitis and asthma are likely to cause breathing difficulties (rapid breathing, increased effort with each breath) over and above the wheeze.

Less common causes of wheezing include feeding difficulties and heart disease.

DID YOU KNOW?

WHEEZING VS. CONGESTION

The noise characteristic of wheezing is different from the noises made by congested nasal passages. Wheezing is typically heard when breathing out (exhaling), while nasal congestion can lead to snoring or noise while breathing in. Wheezing is often accompanied by more rapid and labored breathing than normal, which is not usually the case with nasal congestion.

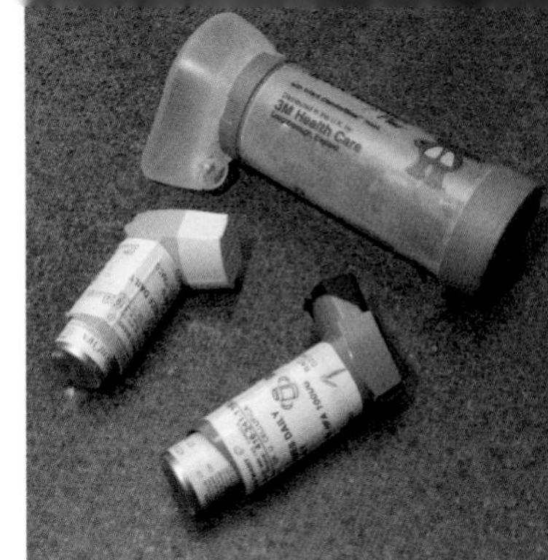

Treating Wheezing

Any infant with signs of breathing difficulty (rapid breathing, increased effort needed to breathe) should be seen immediately by a physician. Because wheezing has a number of causes, your physician may recommend some tests. In a clinic or hospital setting, a monitor can be attached to a finger or toe to check the oxygen level of the blood. An x-ray of the chest will sometimes be warranted.

Bronchiolitis is a self-resolving condition that improves over a period of days. Infants who need more supportive care (oxygen and fluids to prevent dehydration) will require hospitalization. For infants with repeated episodes of wheezing who are suspected to have asthma, your health-care provider may prescribe medications (bronchodilators) administered through a compressor or puffer and spacer device to reverse obstruction to airflow, as well as medication to reduce inflammation of the airways (steroid medication in an inhaled or oral form).

Coughs

The lungs are made up of many tiny branching airways, and a cough is usually an airway's reflex response to irritation. Most coughs are caused by fairly harmless and self-limited viral illnesses, but some can be a sign of a more serious condition that may need specific therapy and urgent attention.

▷ Coughing Red Flags

Seek immediate medical treatment for any of the following signs or symptoms:

- Your baby is having trouble breathing even when not coughing. Breathing difficulties may include rapid or labored breathing.
- The cough is associated with wheezing.
- The cough is associated with a "whoop" or your baby's lips turn blue during a coughing spell.
- The cough occurs after a choking episode and doesn't settle down quickly. This suggests that your baby has aspirated a foreign material (food or toy) into his lungs.
- The cough is associated with fever, vomiting, or listlessness, and your baby is not his normal self.
- The cough is not getting better after a week, or is worrying you for any reason.

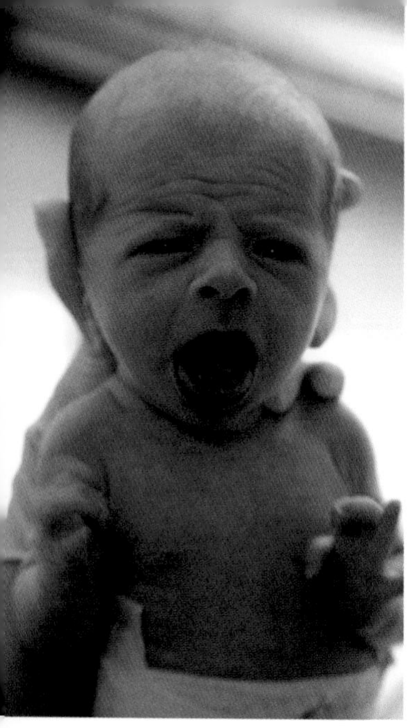

Croup

Croup is a viral infection that causes a loud, barking, seal-like cough. Croup is more common in the spring and fall, and usually follows a few days of cold symptoms. The virus causes inflammation and swelling in the voice box and windpipe (larynx and trachea), leading to the characteristic cough and sometimes to noisy and labored breathing. The cough tends to be most severe in the middle of the night.

Treating Croup

While croup's noisy cough can be frightening, if your child is otherwise breathing comfortably and quietly between bouts of coughing, the croup is classified as mild. Any child who is having difficulty breathing, however, needs to be seen immediately by a physician. Inhaled medications to reduce the swelling in the windpipe will often be used. A dose of oral steroid medication is also given to help reduce the inflammation. Most children recover quickly, but loud coughing can persist for days.

Croup Red Flags

Children with the following signs of breathing difficulty should be assessed in the emergency department of your local hospital:

- A high-pitched noise can be heard when your child inhales (known as stridor).
- Your child appears anxious.
- He is having difficulty swallowing.
- He is obviously using his chest muscles to breathe.

KEY POINT

If a cough settles quickly, there is usually nothing to worry about, but if it continues or your baby experiences any breathing difficulty, wheezing or stridor (a high-pitched noise heard when breathing in), seek medical attention immediately.

Whooping Cough (Pertussis)

If the coughing comes in fits, followed by a whoop or vomiting, or your baby's lips turn blue during a coughing spell, he could have whooping cough. While incompletely immunized and unimmunized children are at much higher risk, even fully immunized babies may still get whooping cough on the odd occasion, although it is likely to be less severe.

If you suspect that your baby may have whooping cough, consult your doctor immediately, especially if he is under 6 months of age.

Choking

It is not unusual for liquids to go down "the wrong way," causing a bit of a choke and a cough. Prevent choking episodes by keeping choking hazards away from your baby and cutting foods into pieces small enough that they can't plug the airway.

Vomiting

Almost every infant vomits at some point. Vomiting should be distinguished from spitting up, or reflux, a normal, effortless regurgitation of stomach contents that occurs most often during and after feeding. Vomiting is a forceful expulsion of stomach contents. Babies may vomit through the nose as well as the mouth. While it certainly isn't pretty, vomiting through the nose does not mean the condition is more severe.

KEY POINT

If you notice a decrease in the amount of urine in your baby's diapers and he is becoming listless and has a dry tongue, sunken eyes, and decreased tears, seek medical attention immediately.

Causes of Vomiting

Infants, and children in general, are more prone to vomiting than adults, and they can vomit for a wide variety of reasons. For example, babies tend to vomit if they have a forceful cough. The most common cause of vomiting is an acute infection, such as a viral intestinal infection or a urinary tract infection. Other causes of vomiting include allergy to milk and obstructions to the stomach and intestinal tract.

Dehydration

Whatever the cause, if your child is vomiting persistently, he may become dehydrated due to the loss of fluids from the stomach. The younger he is, the more quickly he will become dehydrated if he cannot keep fluids down. If he is breast-feeding, continue feeding him normally. If he is formula-fed or on solids, consider supplementing with an oral rehydration solution, available at most drugstores. Small amounts (1 to 2 tsp/5 to 10 mL) given every 5 to 10 minutes seem to work best. The solution can be given by syringe, spoon, bottle, or cup, depending on what your baby is willing to take. Introduce his regular diet once he appears to be adequately rehydrated.

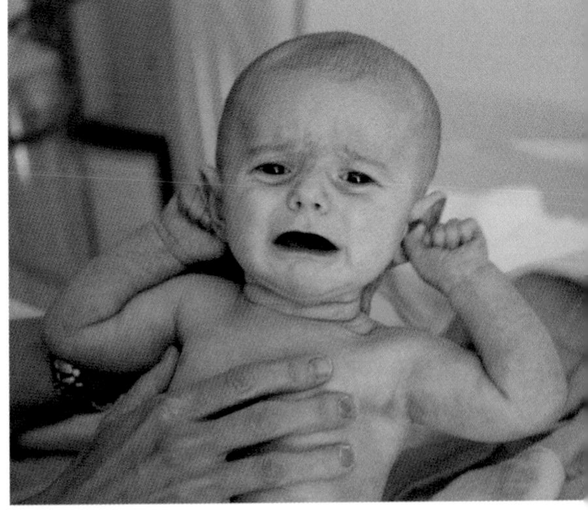

▷ Vomiting Red Flags

Be alert for these red flag signs and symptoms that require urgent medical attention.

- The vomit contains blood, whether fresh blood (this is very unusual) or tiny bits of digested blood that resemble coffee grounds.
- The vomit contains bile. Bile is dark green (not yellow) and could indicate an intestinal obstruction.
- The vomit (particularly in the first 2 months of life) is projectile, traveling up to 3 feet (1 m). This suggests an obstruction at the outlet of the stomach, called pyloric stenosis.
- Your baby has a dry mouth or is not wetting his diapers. These signs could indicate dehydration.
- Your baby is listless and is not interested in feeding or his environment. This indicates dehydration or an infection.
- The vomiting is persistent and your baby is unable to keep anything down.

Managing Vomiting

If your child has vomited just once and looks fine afterwards, continue with normal care. Vomiting that doesn't recur is unlikely to be a cause for concern. If the vomiting recurs, you'll need to determine the cause and follow the treatment procedures for that condition.

Gastroesophageal Reflux

Many young babies spit up on a fairly regular basis due to gastroesophageal reflux. Some babies even vomit forcefully an hour or two after finishing their feed. If this has been happening for weeks or months but your baby seems contented and has continued to gain weight and develop appropriately, intervention is not likely to be necessary; nevertheless, you should mention the persistent vomiting to your health-care provider. If your baby is not gaining weight or seems uncomfortable when feeding (as though he is experiencing heartburn), contact your health-care provider without delay. There are a number of interventions that will improve gastroesophageal reflux. This recurrent condition tends to get better as your child gets older.

Gastroenteritis

Is there an associated change in your baby's stools? The second most common cause of vomiting in infancy is viral gastroenteritis. See page 202 for details.

Infection

Is the vomiting accompanied by other signs of an infection? For example, is your baby lethargic or crying when passing urine? A change in the smell or color of the urine may suggest a urinary tract infection, although dehydration can also make the urine darker and smell a bit "stronger."

A baby who has a fever, is inconsolable, or is listless and "not himself" may have a serious infection, such as meningitis. If he is coughing and having trouble breathing, the vomiting may be a result of pneumonia or bronchiolitis. (It is not unusual for a baby to empty his stomach as part of a forceful cough.) In either case, see your health-care provider immediately.

Intestinal Obstruction

If the vomit is dark green (bile-stained), rather than bright yellow, see your health-care provider immediately. Your baby's bowel may be blocked. Although it is very unusual, intestinal obstruction can occur in healthy infants when a loop of bowel becomes twisted (volvulus) or telescopes into the segment in front of it (intussusception).

Pyloric Stenosis

If the vomiting is projectile, traveling up to 3 feet (1 m), your baby may have an obstruction at the end of the stomach, a condition called pyloric stenosis. It is usually seen in the first 2 months of life, particularly in boys and in babies with a family history of this condition. The vomiting tends to get worse over the course of days, to the point where nothing stays down.

Food Allergies

Allergies to specific foods are quite common in infants. Perhaps the most common is an allergy to cow's milk protein, which can affect both formula-fed and breast-fed babies (a mother who is ingesting dairy products passes the protein on to her baby in her breast milk). Although diarrhea is the most common symptom, vomiting may also result. In addition, you may see blood in the stool, irritability, and poor weight gain. Discuss these symptoms with your health-care provider.

DID YOU KNOW?

BLOOD IN THE VOMIT

Is there blood in your baby's vomit? Blood can look bright red, or darkish purple if clotted. Once it has been in the stomach for a while and is a bit digested, it resembles coffee grounds. There are several ways that blood might get into the stomach: it is not unusual for the stomach lining to ooze blood when inflamed or irritated (gastritis); the lining of the esophagus may become inflamed in babies with gastroesophageal reflux and can be torn slightly by forceful vomiting; and breast-fed babies can swallow blood while feeding if the mother's nipples are cracked or raw. There is no need to panic if you see small quantities of blood, though you should report it to your health-care provider as soon as possible.
If you see lots of fresh blood, seek immediate medical attention.

Gastroenteritis ("Stomach Flu")

A self-limited episode of vomiting and diarrhea (that is, an episode that resolves on its own) is common in young children, usually due to viral intestinal infections (gastroenteritis), which are most prevalent in the winter months. These viruses are hardy (living on tabletops and objects for several days) and very contagious, spreading easily among children in daycare and among family members. Wash your hands carefully after changing your baby's diaper.

Viral intestinal infections can cause fever, vomiting, cramping, loss of appetite, and frequent, watery stools. These symptoms may last several days to a week, although the vomiting and fever usually resolve within 48 hours. While most episodes can be managed at home, these infections can be distressing for families (particularly when several individuals are sick at once) and lead to significant time away from school and work, with frequent visits to medical centers and emergency departments.

DID YOU KNOW?

TYPICAL COURSE

The typical course of gastroenteritis begins with 1 to 2 days of vomiting, when it seems as if everything that goes into the stomach comes right back out again. The vomit usually resembles whatever has been ingested, and may become yellow when the stomach is empty. It may be accompanied by a low-grade fever, as well as signs that your baby is not his normal happy and energetic self. As the vomiting starts to settle, diarrhea will likely begin, with an increased number of smelly and very watery stools.

Treating Gastroenteritis

- **Feeding:** Mild episodes of gastroenteritis require no change in diet. Breast-fed infants should continue breast-feeding. The majority of formula-fed infants can continue their usual formula.
- **Rehydration:** Children who have persistent vomiting or are dehydrated should be offered a commercially prepared oral rehydration solution (Pedialyte or Enfalyte, for example). These are available at most drugstores, and no prescription is required. They do tend to have a slightly salty taste, so pick a flavored variety. Other fluids, such as flat pop, juice, tea, rice water, and soup, do not have the appropriate mix of water, sugar, and salt and should not be used to manage dehydration. Rehydration solution should be offered in frequent but small amounts if your child is vomiting: 1 to 3 ounces (30 to 90 mL) per hour in infants under 6 months; 3 to 4 ounces (90 to 125 mL) per hour in babies 6 to 18 months.
- **Medication:** Acetaminophen (Tylenol, Tempra) can be used if your child appears to have tummy cramps or the fever seems to be bothering him. Consider giving it as a suppository if he can't keep anything down.

- **Medical care:** Children who exhibit signs of complications should be seen by a doctor. While small amounts of blood in the stool can infrequently occur, large amounts suggest a bacterial infection.

▷ Gastroenteritis Red Flags

The major risk to children with intestinal infections is dehydration – the loss of water and salts from excessive vomiting or diarrhea. While mild dehydration can be managed at home, more significant dehydration can be dangerous and must be treated in a hospital.

Watch for these signs:

- Your child is listless and lacks interest in his surroundings.
- He is not wetting his diapers (urine may be difficult to differentiate from watery diarrhea).
- His mouth is dry, without saliva.
- His eyes are sunken or the soft spot (fontanel) in his skull feels very sunken in.
- He cannot keep fluids down.

Constipation

Concern about a baby's stools is one of the most common reasons for parents to seek advice from health-care providers. Many parents worry that their infant is constipated when he is passing fewer stools than they expect. However, there is a wide range of normal stooling patterns during infancy, and the frequency of stools is not a cause for concern as long as they are soft. Constipation is characterized by the passage of hard, painful stools, often in the form of little pellets. Rarely, constipation may be caused by an underlying medical problem.

Treating Constipation

Every well-meaning health-care provider and relative will have suggestions for treating constipation. Simple dietary changes, such as substituting barley for rice cereal and adding 1 to 2 ounces (30 to 60 mL) of prunes to the diet, are sometimes sufficient. Polyethylene glycol 3350 (Miralax, Lax-A-Day) or Lactulose, a non-absorbable sugar similar to prune juice, may be prescribed as a treatment for constipation.

Mineral oil should be avoided during infancy because it can cause a serious form of pneumonia if aspirated into

DID YOU KNOW?

STRAINING

When their baby strains and becomes red in the face while passing stools, many parents interpret this as a sign of constipation. But infants cannot coordinate relaxation of the pelvic muscles with pushing to evacuate the bowels. Straining is the result. If the passed stool is soft, you can usually be reassured that your baby is not constipated. If the stool is hard or a fissure develops, stool softeners may be necessary.

the lungs, and honey and corn syrup should not be used because of the risk of botulism. Regular stimulation of the rectum with fingers, thermometers, or suppositories is not recommended.

Rashes

Skin rashes come in all forms, from raised bumps to flat blotches. Most are transient and harmless. Occasionally, a rash can be a sign of a serious condition (for example, an infection) that needs immediate attention.

Causes of Rashes

Rashes can result from a multitude of causes:

- Transient skin conditions common in early infancy
- Chronic skin conditions (such as eczema and seborrheic dermatitis)
- Allergies
- Infections
- Irritants to the skin (such as diaper dermatitis from contact with urine and stool)

Rash Red Flags

See your health-care provider if your baby's rash has the following characteristics and your baby appears generally unwell:

- The rash is non-blanching (when you press on the skin, the rash does not fade), particularly when accompanied by fever. This type of rash is caused by bleeding into the tissues below the skin and can appear as flat reddish pinpoints or larger purplish bumps. It can sometimes be a sign of a serious infection or a deficiency of platelets in the blood.
- The rash looks infected (it is red, hot, swollen, and painful or is red, oozing, and has a yellow crust).
- Hives — raised pink welts — are present. Hives can be a sign of an allergy to foods, medications, inhaled allergens, or something in contact with the skin. Hives can also be caused by common childhood viruses.

Transient Skin Conditions

Many rashes commonly seen in babies require no intervention. See page 35 for descriptions of milia, baby acne, and erythema toxicum, which may affect your baby's skin as early as the first day of life. Your health-care provider can help you recognize these rashes, as well as heat rash and roseola.

Heat Rash

Heat rash (sometimes called prickly heat) is often seen in young infants when the pores of the sweat glands get plugged. Although most common in hot, humid environments, it may develop in cooler temperatures if the baby is overbundled. Blockage of the pores causes tiny pink-red bumps to develop; they are most prevalent on covered parts of the skin, especially on the upper back and chest.

Heat rash does not cause fever. It usually settles on its own and can be prevented by using cotton clothing that allows heat and moisture to escape, avoiding overbundling, and reducing exposure to excessive heat and humidity.

KEY POINT

Ointments, creams, and powders are not useful in treating heat rash because they can block pores and cause further rash.

Roseola

Roseola is a viral infection caused by human herpes virus 6 (different from the herpes simplex virus that causes cold sores). Roseola characteristically causes a blanching, flat, and slightly raised pinkish rash that typically, though not always, occurs after a few days of fever. The fever generally disappears by the time the rash is apparent, and the rash usually lasts only 1 to 2 days. Three-quarters of children will experience this infection by 1 year of age, most often between 6 and 9 months.

Roseola is self-limited and resolves on its own without any specific treatment, though medications such as acetaminophen or ibuprofen can be used for fever and discomfort.

Eczema

Eczema (atopic dermatitis), which is characterized by patches of red, raised, dry, scaly, and itchy skin, is one of the most common rashes, affecting up to 10% of people. Approximately 60% of people who have eczema develop signs in the first year of life. Eczema is particularly common in families with a history of allergic conditions (asthma, food allergies, and hay fever).

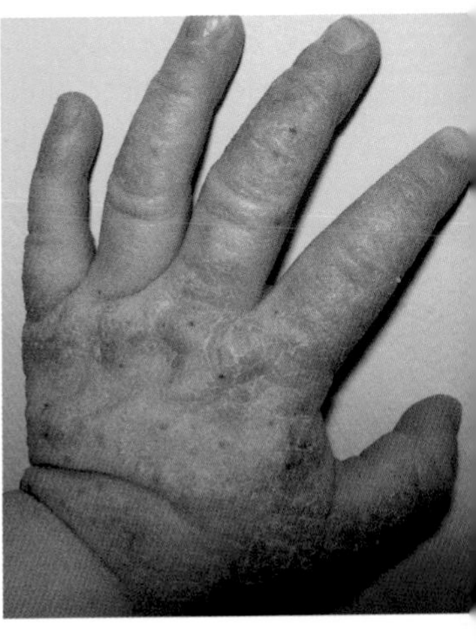

Infants are usually affected on the face, especially the cheeks, although the outside of the knees and elbows can also be involved. The diaper area is typically not involved. While eczema resolves by school age in about 50% of children, 25% of individuals continue to be affected into adulthood.

There are no available treatments that prevent or cure eczema, but there are effective measures to manage the symptoms. Irritants to the skin (harsh soaps, fabric softener, bubble baths) should be avoided, while gentle soaps for infants (such as Baby Dove) and bath moisturizers (such as Aveeno) are helpful. The skin can be kept lubricated with petroleum jelly, which helps to trap moisture in the skin. Your physician will advise you on the use of topical steroid creams or ointments for inflamed areas.

DID YOU KNOW?

ANTIBIOTICS

It is very common for a rash to appear while a baby is taking antibiotics (although it does not usually take the form of hives). This does not necessarily mean that your baby is allergic to that antibiotic. When a viral illness is mistakenly treated with an antibiotic, the appearance of a rash is often related to the natural progression of the viral illness; the antibiotic is just an innocent bystander. Ask your doctor whether your baby is still able to take that antibiotic if needed in the future.

Seborrheic Dermatitis

Seborrheic dermatitis is a common rash that usually develops during the first 3 months of life. When the scalp is involved, it is called cradle cap. Other areas typically affected include the skin over the eyebrows, behind the ears, on the neck, and in the folds in the diaper region. The rash appears as a scaly yellow eruption with reddened, greasy skin often appearing around or under the scales. It is not usually itchy.

Seborrheic dermatitis is typically self-limited and does not require treatment. In fact, baby oils often exacerbate the condition. Anti-seborrheic shampoos can be used for more extensive, cosmetically bothersome, or inflamed scalp eruptions. Used three to four times a week, the shampoo is left on for approximately 5 minutes, followed by gentle combing of the scales. Vigorous removal of the scales should not be attempted. A mild topical steroid medication may also be advised by your physician for inflamed areas.

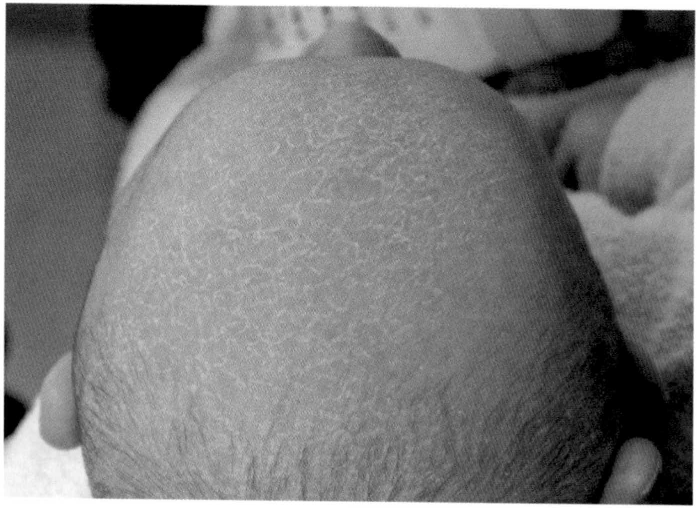

Seborrheic dermatitis

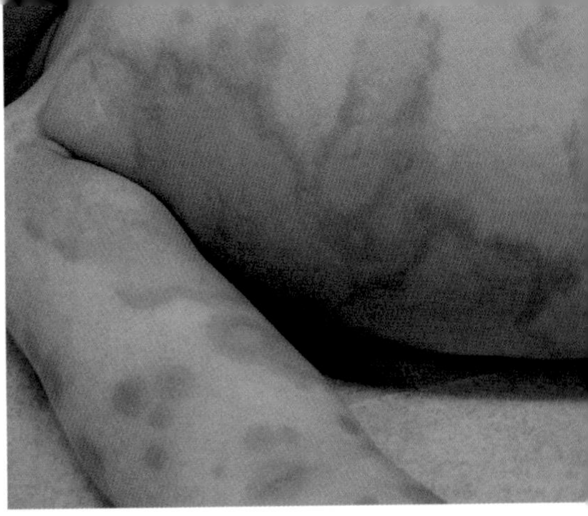

Allergic Reactions

Less commonly, allergic reactions can cause a rash in infants. Hives can be a sign of an allergic reaction to foods, medications, inhaled allergens (animal dander), or something in contact with the skin. Hives appear as raised pink-red welts; they usually appear and disappear within hours and are generally itchy. If the cause of the reaction is clear, remove the allergen.

Viral Infections

If, in addition to a rash, your baby has a fever or cold symptoms, is feeding poorly, or is irritable, the rash is likely related to a viral infection, especially if it is a non-specific, pinkish, generally flat rash that blanches when pressure is applied. This type of rash can occur anywhere on the body. How quickly you seek medical attention depends on how unwell your baby looks.

Diaper Rash

The diaper area is a prime target for rashes because it is warm and moist. In addition, the delicate skin under the diaper is exposed to lots of irritating urine and feces. You can prevent diaper rashes by changing your baby's diaper frequently (at least every 2 hours), applying a barrier cream with diaper changes, and avoiding the use of harsh soaps and detergents.

The most common form of diaper rash is diaper dermatitis (inflammation of the skin in the diaper area). It begins as red, inflamed skin, does not involve the skin folds, and can lead to raw, open areas of skin.

The yeast *Candida albicans* is another common culprit, especially if your baby has been recently treated with antibiotics. Antibiotics, in addition to getting rid of harmful bacteria, tend to kill off some of the good germs that usually compete with yeasts, thereby allowing the yeasts to flourish and giving rise to thrush and candida diaper rash. This rash looks bright red, with small red blotches beyond the margins (satellite lesions). Unlike diaper dermatitis, a yeast rash involves the folds between the chubby rolls of skin. Suspect a yeast rash if it does not respond to regular treatment and involves the folds.

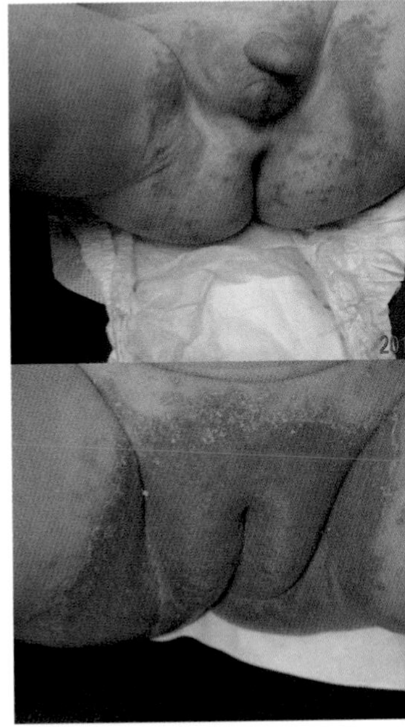

TOP: Irritant diaper rash
BOTTOM: Candida diaper rash

HOW TO: Treat Diaper Rash

Diaper Dermatitis

- Change diapers frequently and gently cleanse the area with a cloth soaked in warm water. Remember that this type of rash is caused by irritants (urine and stool) on the skin, so removing them from the skin is at least as important as putting creams on it.
- Use a thick layer of barrier paste, which usually contains zinc oxide in varying strengths. The barrier keeps the urine and stool off the irritated skin and should be applied with every diaper change.
- See your doctor if the rash does not improve after a few days or involves skin breakdown. Sometimes a mild topical steroid ointment is needed.

Candida Rash

- This rash is usually easily treated with antifungal ointments prescribed by your doctor.

Oral Thrush

Babies with candida rash sometimes also have oral thrush, a yeast infection in the mouth. It looks like a thick white plaque on the tongue or elsewhere inside the mouth. Nearly one-third of all infants will develop oral thrush.

Oral thrush can cause pain with eating. The surface of the tongue or cheeks may be raw and may bleed slightly if you attempt to remove the thrush. However, most infants are not bothered by it. Thrush does not usually interfere with feeding, nor does it cause a fever.

Preventing Oral Thrush

To prevent oral thrush, place bottle nipples and pacifiers in boiling water for 5 to 10 minutes, or wash them in the dishwasher. Make sure to cool them before your baby uses them. Hand-washing is also important.

DID YOU KNOW?

BREAST-FEEDING MOTHERS

If you are breast-feeding, be sure to get treated for thrush yourself. Breast-feeding mothers can develop itchy, crusty, burning nipples due to a thrush infection (see the table on page 68). Yeast infections can be passed back and forth from mother's nipples to baby's mouth.

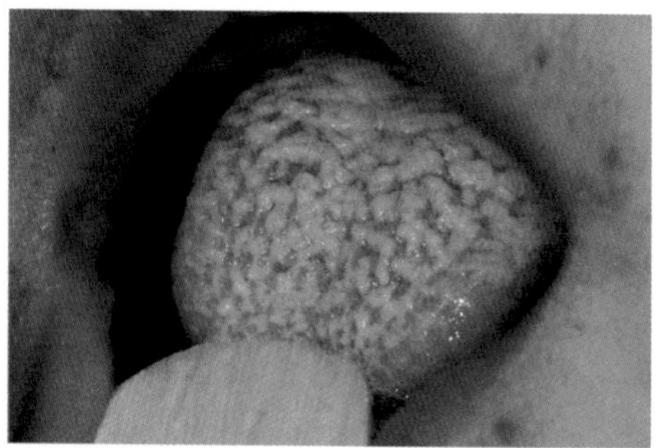

Treating Oral Thrush

Your baby's doctor can prescribe a medication called nystatin, which is painted onto the plaques in the baby's mouth four times daily for about 1 week. Most oral thrush will clear up within a few days of starting nystatin. For more resistant cases, see the doctor for reassessment.

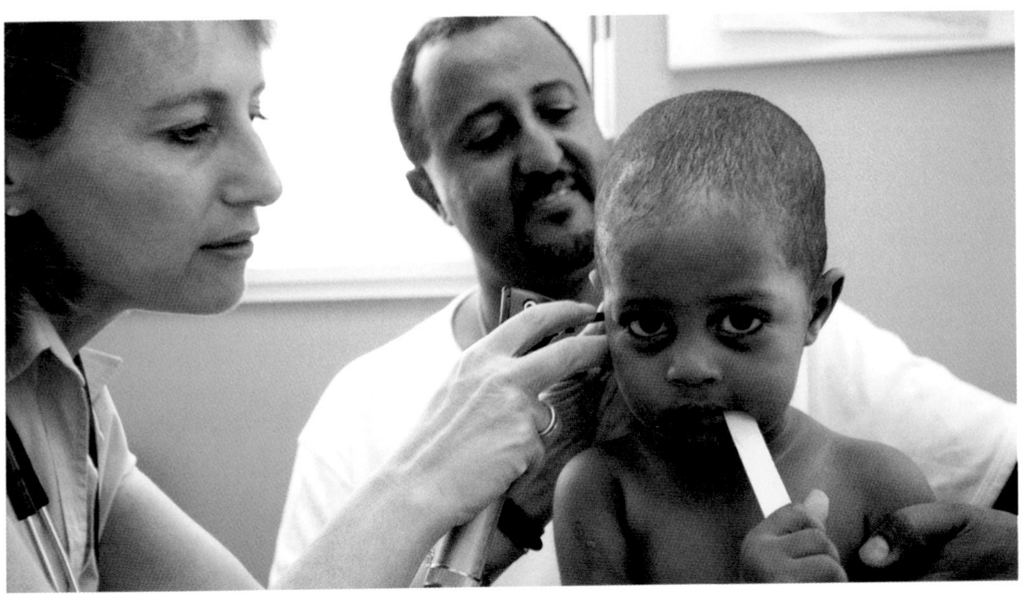

Ear Infections

One of the most common infections (and reasons for antibiotic use) in young children is otitis media, an infection of the middle ear (the small space behind the eardrum). The majority of children will have had at least one ear infection by the time they are 2 to 3 years old. Young infants, usually starting at around 6 months of age, are particularly prone to these infections. They pick up a number of cold viruses, which lead to upper respiratory infections and may result in a buildup of fluid behind the eardrum that cannot drain due to a blocked eustachian tube. This fluid becomes a fertile place for bacteria and viruses to multiply and produce an infection.

Diagnosing Ear Infections

Most ear infections follow a common cold. Some signs that an ear infection is present include fever, fussiness, and ear rubbing or pulling. Infants with ear infections may often have difficulty sleeping.

Your doctor will confirm the diagnosis of an ear infection, using an instrument called an otoscope to look for redness, pus, swelling, or a perforation in the eardrum.

Treating Ear Infections

Most ear infections, especially in older children, will resolve on their own within a few days without any treatment, but an oral antibiotic may be prescribed for children under

2 years of age with persistent or severe symptoms, or if the ear drum is perforated. Medications for pain and fever, such as acetaminophen (Tylenol, Tempra) or ibuprofen (Advil, Motrin), are usually recommended to keep your child comfortable.

DID YOU KNOW?

VENTILATING TUBES

Fluid in the middle ear often takes weeks to drain. Rarely, some children will have a persistent buildup of fluid, which can interfere with hearing. If fluid buildup is present for more than several months, your doctor might discuss putting tiny ventilating tubes in the eardrums, a simple operation performed by an ear, nose, and throat surgeon. This short procedure is usually done as day surgery. Ventilating tubes are also inserted if your child's hearing is affected or infections recur frequently.

Eye Discharge

Tears drain through small ducts in the inner corners of the lower eyelids, called the lacrimal ducts, or tear ducts. These ducts drain into the top part of the nose, which explains why your nose often runs when you have a good cry! Some babies, however, are born with blocked or narrowed tear ducts, on one or both sides. These babies may often look teary even if they are happy.

Babies with blocked tear ducts sometimes have a collection of milky yellow discharge in the inner corner of their eyes. Occasionally, a baby will not be able to open his eye because the lids are stuck together with the crusty material. Parents often mistake this as a sign of an eye infection. If the white parts of your baby's eyes are not red and there aren't copious amounts of thick pus, the problem is likely just a blocked tear duct or ducts.

Treating Eye Discharge

Wet a clean washcloth or gauze and use it to wipe away the crusty material. If the duct is still blocked, apply gentle

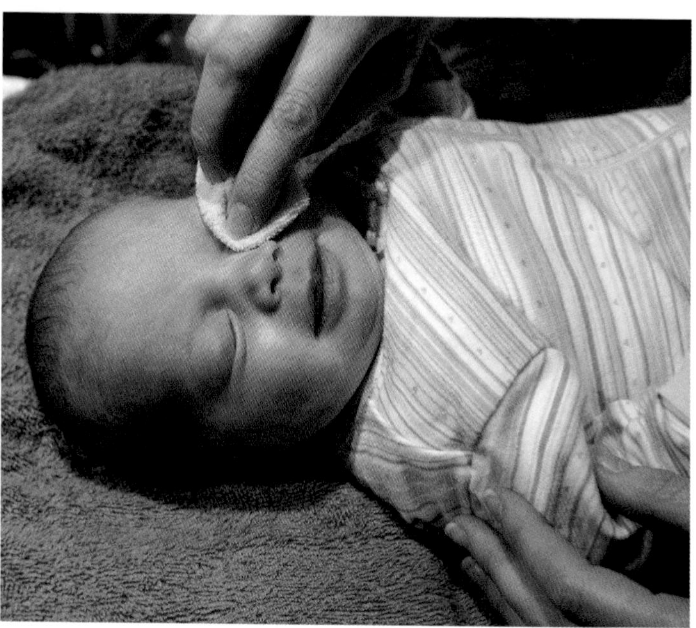

pressure along the nose and underneath the eye several times a day. Ask your health-care provider how to do this.

Giving Medicine to Your Baby

As many parents can attest, the decision to give medication, such as acetaminophen for fever or antibiotics for an ear infection, may be straightforward, but actually administering the medication to a baby can be far from easy.

Some medications are best given orally, by dropper or syringe. Others can be given by rectal suppository; this route is most helpful when your child is vomiting. Medicines can take 30 to 45 minutes to be absorbed or to pass through the stomach. If your child vomits within 15 to 30 minutes of being given an oral medication, the dose can be repeated.

Infant Medications

Medications can be divided into those purchased over the counter (OTC) and those that are prescribed. For a list of some of the OTC and prescribed medications commonly used in the first year of life, see the chart on page 213.

Almost all medications have the potential for unwanted side effects. While many are of minor importance, in rare circumstances more serious adverse effects, such as a severe allergic reaction, can result.

Oral Administration (by Dropper or Syringe)

- Shake the bottle before use.
- Carefully check the dosage recommendations on the label. It is very easy to mix up mL and mg, and different formulations of antipyretics, for example, may have different strengths.
- Use a dropper or syringe to get the medicine into your baby's mouth. Place the tip of the dropper or syringe in his mouth so that the tip is pointing toward the cheek and slowly squeeze the dropper or press the syringe plunger.
- To help prevent gagging, avoid squirting liquid medication at the roof of the mouth or the back of the tongue. Small squirts into the space between the gum and cheek often work best. It will also be harder for your infant to spit out the medicine this way.
- Check the storage directions. Some liquid medications, such as antibiotics, need to be stored in the refrigerator.

KEY POINT

Side effects are not limited to prescribed medications; they can also be caused by over-the-counter medications, as well as naturopathic and herbal remedies. When you're deciding whether to give your infant a medication, it is always wise to weigh the risks and benefits.

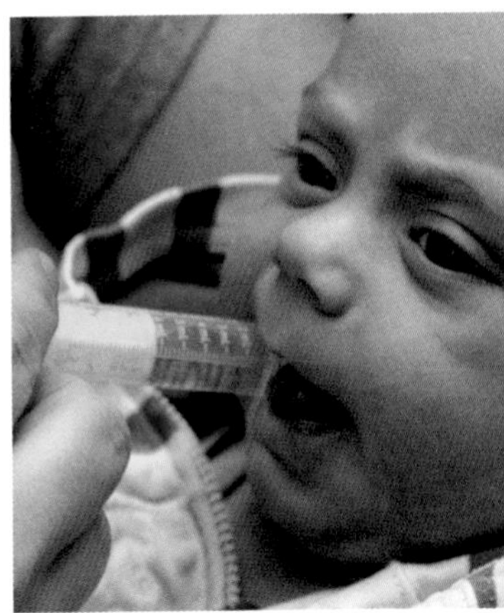

KEY POINT

Caution should be used when using syringes that come with caps on the end to prevent spillage — these small caps can be a choking hazard.

Rectal Administration (by Suppository)

- Lie your baby on his back.
- Place your baby's hips and knees in a flexed position to relax the anus and make administration easier.
- Insert the suppository gently into the anus using a small amount of petroleum jelly as a lubricant.

HOW TO: Give Eye, Nose, and Ear Drops

Infections involving the eyes, ears, and nose are not uncommon in infants. While it may be difficult to get the drops into these sensitive (and small) parts of the body, drops are often safer and more effective than other forms of administration because the medication goes directly to the site of the infection. In addition, because only a minimal amount is absorbed into the bloodstream, the risk of side effects is lower.

Eye Drops

- Warm the bottle in your hands.
- Wrap your baby in a blanket.
- Lay your baby on his back and gently pull his lower eyelid down with your thumb, forming a pocket for the drops.
- If your baby resists opening his eyes, drop the liquid onto the inner corner of the eye and rub gently with your fingertip. As your baby opens his eyes, the medication will be absorbed.
- Never touch the eye with the dropper.

Nose Drops

- Warm the bottle in your hands.
- Wrap your baby in a blanket.
- Lay your baby on his back so that his head falls back over your thigh, and support his head with your hand.
- Place the tip of the dropper just above the nostril and give the drops as prescribed.

Ear Drops

- Warm the bottle in your hands.
- Wrap your baby in a blanket.
- Lay your baby on his side on your lap, with his infected ear facing up.
- Gently pull his earlobe down and back to straighten the ear canal.
- Drop, don't squirt, drops into ear.
- Keep your baby lying down for a minute to prevent the drops from running out.

Infant Medications

NAME	INDICATIONS	EXAMPLES	DOSE	COMMENTS
Antipyretics and analgesics	• Fever • Discomfort	• Acetaminophen (Tylenol, Tempra) • Ibuprofen (Advil, Motrin)	• 10–15 mg per kg every 4–6 hours or consult package • *Under 6 months:* 5 mg per kg every 8 hours as necessary • *Over 6 months:* 5–10 mg per kg every 6 to 8 hours as necessary	• Do not use in babies under 3 months unless discussed with your doctor.
Antibiotics	• Bacterial infections: for example, ear infections, urinary tract infections, skin infections, pneumonia	• Amoxicillin	• 50–90 mg per kg daily (usually given in three divided doses), depending on the indication for use	• Different types of antibiotics are required depending on the type of infection and the causative bacteria. • Complete the full course of antibiotics to avoid breeding resistant bacteria.
Laxatives	• Constipation	• Glycerin suppository • Lactulose • Polyethylene glycol 3350	• 1 infant suppository as necessary • ½–1 tsp (2.5–5 mL) daily or twice daily • 1 g per kg daily	• Constipation in babies less than 6 months should be evaluated by your health-care provider prior to starting treatment.
Topical creams and ointments	• Eczema • Fungal infections	• 1% hydrocortisone cream • Nystatin ointment	• Apply three times daily to affected area	• Only mild steroid creams and ointments should be used on the face and diaper area. • Ointments are preferred to creams.

Frequently Asked Questions

Should I get something at the drugstore for my baby's cold?

Dozens of over-the-counter medications marketed as treatments for cold symptoms are available. Apart from medications that relieve discomfort and fever, such as acetaminophen and ibuprofen, these products have not been shown to benefit young infants and children and, in many situations, can cause unwanted or harmful side effects. In general, avoid these products for children under school age.

My mother told me to feed a cold and starve a fever. Is this true for babies?

Absolutely not – and it's not true for adults, either. When a baby is unwell, whether with a cold or a fever, it is important that she remain well hydrated, so offer lots of liquids. Most babies lose their appetite when sick, but you should continue to offer them their regular foods – just don't be disappointed if they aren't eating as well as usual.

If the prescription says to give my son his antibiotic every 6 hours, should I wake him to take the dose?

Very few medications must be given exactly every 6 or 8 hours. If your son is sick, you both likely need your sleep. In the case of antibiotics and most other medications, it would be reasonable to give him a dose before he goes to sleep, and, if you are lucky enough that he sleeps for 7 or 8 hours, give him the next dose when he wakes up.

My daughter is 6 months old. How should I be taking her temperature? I used to use a glass/mercury thermometer. Are the newer digital ones better?

A child has to be about 4 to 5 years old before you are likely to get an accurate result by taking her temperature orally. Ear thermometers are expensive and are not particularly accurate for children under 2 years. Rectal thermometers are the most accurate, but most children do not appreciate having their temperature taken rectally, so it is usually reserved for babies under 3 months, for whom an accurate temperature reading is more important. For a 6-month-old, we suggest taking her temperature under her arm.

We prefer digital thermometers because they read the temperature much more quickly, so you don't have to hold your child down for long. With glass thermometers, there is always a risk, albeit very slight, that it will break – and the mercury inside is toxic.

I've heard a lot about the dangers of the flu. My baby is almost 1 month old now — should I be getting him vaccinated against it?

The current vaccine available for influenza can only be used from 6 months of age onward. If your baby will be over 6 months old in October or November, when it is time for the annual influenza vaccination, it is advisable to have him immunized. Otherwise, all caregivers and other household contacts should be vaccinated to reduce the likelihood that your baby becomes exposed to influenza.

Baby Care Resources

We have witnessed a dramatic transformation in the way people learn about things. The Internet and sophisticated search engines, such as "Doctor" Google, have put vast amounts of information at the disposal of millions of people. Simply pick a topic, and thousands of websites pertaining to a given subject become immediately available. We are now capable of informing just about everyone about pretty well everything.

But people can get misinformation on the Internet just as easily. There is no requirement demanding that websites be screened for accuracy. Opinion can replace fact. What you read on any subject may or may not be either authoritative or true.

What, then, is a parent seeking advice to do when trying to filter all the available information? The solution is to seek answers from websites sponsored by well-respected professional health or educational organizations and official government agencies. The advice on these websites is carefully researched and written. Even so, trust your instincts: any advice you are given should make sense to you, regardless of the source.

Here is a short list of reliable North American resources. However, your child's health-care providers remain your best source of information.

Parenting Corner
American Academy of Pediatrics (AAP)
www.healthychildren.org
Authoritative information in an American context.

Caring for Kids
Canadian Paediatric Society (CPS)
www.caringforkids.cps.ca
Authoritative information in a Canadian context.

American College of Obstetricians and Gynecologists
www.acog.org/Patients
Best source for information on pregnancy and childbirth in an American context.

Society of Obstetricians and Gynaecologists of Canada
sogc.org/womens-health-information
Best source for information on pregnancy and childbirth in a Canadian context.

National Institute of Child Health and Human Development
www.nichd.nih.gov
Official site of the U.S. government office on children's health.

Canadian Institute of Child Health
www.cich.ca
An advocate for children's health in a Canadian context.

About Kids Health
The Hospital for Sick Children
www.aboutkidshealth.ca
Comprehensive source of practical guidelines for baby and child care.

Acknowledgments

We would like to express our sincere gratitude to a number of individuals who have helped make this book possible. Creating a book like this is really a team effort!

First and foremost, we would like to acknowledge Norm Saunders, who passed away too soon, some years before this book was realized. Norm was the consummate pediatrician, teacher, mentor, friend, and father. He was a compassionate clinician, a brilliant thinker, and an exceptional communicator. Much of this book is based on his previously written work, and we hope we have done him justice in modeling how he would guide, comfort, and support all of the families he encountered. Norm has left an indelible legacy — a reminder to approach life with dedication, determination, passion, and, most of all, integrity. He continues to inspire us.

Our contributing authors to the original *Baby Care Book* must also be recognized: Sherri Adams, Carolyn Beck, Catherine Birken, Sheila Jacobson, Michelle Shouldice, and Michael Weinstein. Their expertise and contributions to the original writing, upon which this book is based, have been invaluable.

Thank you to the wonderful team at Robert Rose (Bob Dees, Sue Sumeraj, Marian Jarkovich), as well as Kevin Cockburn and his colleagues at PageWave Graphics. As always, this talented and creative group has been easy to work with and has done an outstanding job of presenting the information in a clear, attractive, and practical format for readers.

We would like to thank Denis Daneman, our Pediatrician-in-Chief at SickKids, for his leadership, unwavering support, and commitment to providing the best possible environment for all of us at SickKids to succeed in any endeavor we undertake. Also, a big thanks to Angela McGerrigle for all of her administrative help; and to our SickKids photographers, Diogenes Baena and Robert Teteruck, as well as Dr. Gordon Soon for contributing many of the beautiful photographs that help to bring the pages to life. Thanks also to our many "models," including the children of the contributing authors, other SickKids faculty, and patients.

Finally, a big thank you to our families, Shelley, Sam, and Danielle, and Lynn, Lyndsey, Bethany, Megan, Justin, Nathan, and Hailey, for their endless support and encouragement, and for making raising, and being part of, a family so enormously rewarding.

Photography Credits

All photos by Robert Teteruck, Diogenes Baena and the Dermatology Clinic, © The Hospital for Sick Children, except: **page 3** © iStockphoto.com/iñaki antoñana plaza; **page 5** © iStockphoto.com/IPGGutenbergUKLtd; **page 7** © iStockphoto.com/Aldo Murillo; **page 8** Natasha Saunders; **page 10** © iStockphoto.com/gilaxia; **page 13** © iStockphoto.com/monkeybusinessimages; **page 19** Natasha Saunders; **page 20** Natasha Saunders; **page 23** © iStockphoto.com/crysrob; **page 25** Gordon Soon; **page 27** Gordon Soon; **page 33** Jeremy Friedman; **page 34** Natasha Saunders; **page 35** Natasha Saunders and Gordon Soon; **page 37** Gordon Soon; **page 43** © iStockphoto.com/skynesher; **page 53** Beverly Daniels Photography; **page 55** Natasha Saunders; **page 57** © iStockphoto.com/RuslanDashinsky; **page 82** Gordon Soon; **page 94** Natasha Saunders; **page 97** Natasha Saunders; **page 100** © iStockphoto.com/Dori OConnell; **page 103** © iStockphoto.com/MachineHeadz; **page 105** Natasha Saunders; **page 106** Gordon Soon; **page 107** Natasha Saunders; **page 110** Natasha Saunders; **page 115** Gordon Soon; **page 117** Gordon Soon; **page 118** Natasha Saunders; **page 119** Natasha Saunders; **page 125** Natasha Saunders; **page 127** Jeremy Friedman; **page 140** Natasha Saunders; **page 144** Gordon Soon; **page 154** Natasha Saunders; **page 159** Natasha Saunders; **page 168** © iStockphoto.com/Brian McEntire; **page 171** Natasha Saunders; **page 172** © iStockphoto.com/Floortje; **page 173** Gordon Soon; **page 174** © iStockphoto.com/DMP1; **page 177** © iStockphoto.com/Christopher Futcher; **page 180** © iStockphoto.com/matmart; **page 192** © iStockphoto.com/fredgoldstein; **page 194** © iStockphoto.com/ValuaVitaly; **page 211** Natasha Saunders.

Every effort has been made to contact and obtain permission for the photographs in this book. If omissions and errors have occurred, we encourage you to contact the publisher.

Library and Archives Canada Cataloguing in Publication

Friedman, Jeremy, author

Baby care basics / Dr. Jeremy Friedman, MB, ChB, FRCPC, FAAP; Dr. Natasha Saunders, MD, MSc, FRCPC; with Dr. Norman Saunders, MD, FRCPC.

Includes index.
ISBN 978-0-7788-0519-9 (paperback)

1. Pediatrics—Popular works. 2. Infants—Care—Popular works.
I. Saunders, Norman, author II. Saunders, Natasha, 1979-, author III. Title.

RJ61.F7477 2015 618.92 C2015-903858-8

Index

C

D

E

F

G

H

I

J

K

L

M

N

O

P

R

S

T

U

V

W

X

Y

Z